Refocusing Postgraduate Medical Education:

from the technical to the moral mode of practice

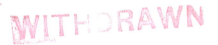
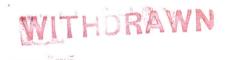

Studies in Education for Medical Practice
Book 1

Refocusing Postgraduate Medical Education:

from the technical to the moral mode of practice

Della Fish

Aneumi **Publications**

Cranham, Gloucester UK

Aneumi Publications
An imprint of ED4MEDPRAC Ltd
A Limited Company: Registration No: 05648049

The Lodge
Cranham Corner
Cranham
GLoucester, UK
GL4 8HB

email: via www.ED4MEDPRAC.co.uk

First published in 2012

A catalogue record of this book is available from the British Library

ISBN:978-0-9572967-0-1

Library of Congress Cataloguing-in-Publication Data
CIP data has been applied for

Cover design and type set in Gill Sans by Jobo Design
www.jobodesign.co.uk

Printed by Severnprint Limited,
8-11 Ashville Trading Estate,
Bristol Road,
Gloucester GL2 5EU
Registered in England: 1317797
www.severnprint.co.uk

Contents

Figures, Frames and Tables   ix
Glossary   x
Acknowledgements   xi
Foreword   xiii

Introduction   3

        Starting with a challenge
        The impact of the current context on medical educational practice
        The argument of this book
        The aims of this book
        The structure of the book
        The readership
        The title

Part One   11
Putting the education back into postgraduate medicine: towards a coherent philosophy

Chapter One   Seeing postgraduate medical education anew: revealing the   13
need for enhanced teaching

        Introduction
        Starting points: the initial details of the investigation
        An analysis and interpretation of the evidence
        Absent themes
        From the traditional to the enhanced approach to teaching
        Enhanced teaching and better patient care
        Starting on the journey
        Further reading

Chapter Two   Seeing our aspirations anew: mapping the journey towards   27
educational *praxis*

        Introduction
        The mountain of educational *praxis*: starting on the pathway
        An overview of the journey
        Aspirations for your journey
        Where this way of thinking comes from: what Aristotle can teach us
        Further reading

Chapter Three   Seeing professional practice anew: exploring the nature   43
of education and medicine

        Introduction
        Clarifying some terms: 'practice' and 'professional practice'
        Rival conceptions of the nature of professional practice
        The nature of practice in medicine and how we might construe it
        The nature of practice in education and how we might construe it
        Modes of practice in education and medicine
        Last words
        Further reading

**Chapter Four   Seeing the teacher's responsibilities anew: a view from the   63
moral mode of practice**

Introduction
Training and education: key differences in teachers' responsibilities
Teaching as a moral activity: what it means to work in the moral mode
of practice
So, in the light of this, what is 'good' teaching?
Further reading

**Chapter Five   Seeing the overall purpose anew: starting from aims and   77
intentions that are properly educational**

Introduction
An overview of the logic of educational aims and intentions
Some key issues about educational aims
Aims arising from the nature of education
Further reading

**Chapter Six   Seeing learners anew: recognizing our moral responsibilities   91
to them**

Introduction
A new role for learners in postgraduate medical and surgical practice
Some important characteristics of postgraduate doctors as learners
Developing the learning doctor as a whole person
Further reading

**Chapter Seven   Seeing educational theory anew: exploring its nature and   103
purpose**

Introduction
An exploration and refutation of some false assumptions
Considering the nature and purpose of educational theory
The main constituents of formal educational theory
Theories that underpin this book's view of learning and teaching
The centrality of language to learning
The vital importance of clinical reflection as central to learning in PGME
Further reading

Chapter Eight   Seeing assessment anew: re-asserting its educational role   119

Introduction
Definitions of assessment
Assessment in the technical mode of practice
Assessment in the moral model of practice
Competence, a competency and competencies
Final comments
Further reading

Part Two   135
The practical implications: how changing understanding changes practice

Chapter Nine   Enriched teaching in medical practice: towards *praxis*   137
    Introduction
    Responsibilities and definitions
    Thinking like an educator: planning for teaching
    Thinking like an educator: methods, content, evaluation and quality
    Developing your own educational philosophy

Chapter Ten   Enriched learning in medical practice: nurturing the learner   159
as a person and clinician
    Introduction
    Studying the learner
    The role of language in learning
    Principles for engaging learners in educational dialogue
    Some principles for improving learning
    Reflection as a central means of learning in and through service

Chapter Eleven   Enriched *informal* assessment: diagnosing where learners   175
are, enabling more focused teaching

    Introduction
    Informal and formal assessments and how they relate to formative and
    summative assessments
    Using informal assessment to study the learner and promote learning
    Some examples of the design of informal assessments
    The quality and use of informal formative assessment
    Endnote

Chapter Twelve   Enriched *formal* assessment: using better teaching and   189
learning to enhance the required 'tools'

    Introduction
    The formal assessment 'tools' for workplace based assessment in PGME
    The Foundation Curriculum (2012) and how it relates to earlier versions
    Making these assessment processes more educational
    The significance of portfolios: some ideas for the future
    Last words

Appendix: A list of the Classical and Thomist virtues   205

References   207

Index   213

Figures, Frames and Tables

Figures

2.1   An overview of the mountain of educational practice   29

2.2   The mountain of educational practice: detail   38

3.1   Understanding modes of practice in medical education: a continuum   60

8.1   Understanding modes of practice in medical education: the role of assessment   132

Frames

1.1   Some important ideas about education not evidenced anywhere during the first observation   18

3.1   Some comments about professionalism   47

5.1   Possible aims for Postgraduate Medical Education (PGME)   80

7.1   Three sample definitions of learning   110

8.1   A definition of assessment   121

9.1   PGME that is 'educationally worthwhile'   141

9.2   Some important issues for planning   145

10.1   Using talk for collective thinking   168

12.1   Educational *praxis* in action   201

Tables

1.1   Towards a shared purpose in PGME for better patient care   23

2.1   Towards educational *praxis*   39

2.2   An Aristotelian classification of *Forms of Reasoning*   40

3.1   Some constituents of the traditions of practice   48

4.1   Some roles that teachers can adopt   68

8.1   The vital distinctions between competence and competencies   128

9.1   Three Models of Teaching   149

9.2   Teaching a procedure: turning training into education   151

Glossary

A & E	Accident and Emergency
ALS	Advanced Life Support
ATLS	Advanced Trauma Life Support
AoME	Academy of Medical Educators
BMA	British Medical Association
CBD	Case Based Discussion
CbDPlus ©	Case-based Discussion Plus Process
CRW	Clinical Reflective Writing
DOPs	Direct Observation of Procedures
E-portfolios	Electronic portfolios
EWTD	European Working Time Directive
F1 doctor	Foundation Doctor, Year One
F2 doctor	Foundation doctor, Year Two
GMC	General Medical Council
GPPS	The General Professional Practice of Surgery
HEE	Health Education England
SLEs	Supervised Learning Events
MDT	Multi-Disciplinary Team
MEE	Medical Education England
Mini-CEX	Mini-Clinical Examination
MMC	Modernising Medical Careers
MSF	Multi-Source Feedback
MTAS	Medical Trainee Application System
NHS	National Health Service
PMETB	Postgraduate Medical Education and Training Board
PG Cert	Postgraduate Certificate
PGME	Postgraduate Medical Education
TAB	Team Assessment of Behaviour
UK	United Kingdom
WPBA	Work Place Based Assessment

Acknowledgements

Firstly, formal thanks are due to Peter de Liefde, founder and owner of **Sense Publications: Rotterdam,** for permission to reprint on pages 151 - 53 the contents of *Table 9.2. Teaching a procedure: turning training into education,* which was first published in J. Higgs, D. Fish, I. Goulter, S. Loftus, J-A. Reid and F. Trede (eds) (2010) *Education for Future Practice.* Rotterdam: Sense Publications, 191 - 202.

Special thanks go to **Professor Michael Thomas,** Pro-Vice Chancellor, University of Chester. I am delighted that he has been willing and able in the time available to write the Foreword, and I also thank him for permission to quote, in the final pages of this book, from the work of nine course members of the Masters Pathway in Education for Postgraduate Medical Practice, (validated by Chester University), whilst their work was still copyright to the university. His support for the educational enterprise that lies behind this book, and for the book itself have been particularly encouraging.

Those course members who appear in person at the end of the book have also contributed various words anonymously to earlier chapters, and have certainly taught me more than I have taught them over the several years we have worked together. They are all very senior clinicians at The Countess of Chester NHS Foundation Trust. In alphabetical order, I thank: **Ann Baker,** Clinical Education Manager; **Dr Ian Benton,** Consultant Respiratory Physician; **Dr Lyndsay Cheater,** Consultant in Anaesthesia and Critical Care Medicine; **Dr Jamie Fanning,** Specialty Doctor in Anaesthetics and Critical Care; **Miss Katharine Fleming,** Consultant in Oral and Maxillofacial Surgery, Regional Maxillofacial Unit, University Hospital, Aintree and the Countess of Chester Hospital; **Dr Eileen Fantom,** Associate Specialist in Emergency Medicine; **Mr Nick Laundy,** Emergency Medicine Consultant and Foundation Training Programme Director; **Dr Natalie Meara,** Consultant Histopathologist; and **Mr David Monk,** Consultant General and Upper Gastrointestinal Surgeon.

Paul Davies at Severnprint Ltd. also deserves much thanks for working with me in producing the graphics associated with The Mountain of Educational Practice as found on the cover and within, and also for seeing this book through the Press.

Without **Jo Richardson of Jobo Design** there would have been nothing to print. I would like to place on record what a privilege it has been to work with someone who is as meticulous and proud about the quality of her work as I try to be about my own. Further, she has gone well beyond the call of duty in helping me to finalize a clean and accurate text. Jo's achievements are the greater for having taken place against the backdrop of some particularly difficult personal times during the book preparation. Consummate professional are the words that come to mind!

Linda de Cossart CBE, Director of Medical Education at The Countess of Chester NHS Foundation Trust, Chester and Visiting Professor at Chester University is another such expert, professional, colleague and friend, without whose support, help and encouragement I could not have begun, let alone completed this work. She has read and advised on many drafts and alongside this has generously and effectively managed the unbelievable amount of backroom and personal support that a project like this demands.

For other contributions to or helpful comments on the contents, I thank: **Professor Jacky Hayden,** Dean of Postgraduate Medical Studies, North Western Deanery and Manchester University; **Dr Martin Talbot,** Consultant in Genito-urinary Medicine/HIV, Honorary University Reader in Medical Education and Academic Directorate of Communicable Diseases, Royal Hallamshire Hospital Sheffield; **Mr Jan Nawrocki,** Consultant Urological Surgeon, Brighton & Sussex University Hospitals NHS Trust and Associate Dean, Kent Surrey & Sussex Deanery; **Dr Clive Weston,** Consultant Physician/Cardiologist, Singleton Hospital,

Swansea, Sub-Dean for Professional Development and Head of Learning & Teaching, College of Medicine, Swansea University; **Dr Gillian Malster**, Retired Consultant Geriatrician and **Renate Thomé**, Clinical Education Consultant and Evaluator.

For keeping me fit to write the book and unwittingly contributing to one of the chapters, I thank **Miss Michelle Lucarotti**, Consultant General and Colorectal Surgeon, Gloucester Royal Hospitals.

I also acknowledge with genuine gratitude **all the consultants and their learners whom I have had the pleasure both to teach and to learn from over the last fourteen years and also all the colleagues with whom I have worked in Postgraduate Medical Education: those in what was South Thames Deanery; those in Kent, Surrey & Sussex Deanery; those in what was the Wessex Deanery; those in the All Wales Deanery and those in the Mersey Deanery.** Because this adds up to considerably more than 400 people, clearly they are too many to name, but they have all certainly left their indelible and important mark on the staging posts of my own journey in understanding Postgraduate Medical Education. They know who they are, and I thank them all.

Last, but by no means least, I thank for their patience, support, encouragement and rigour both **Jean Douglas** and **Evelyn Usher**, who have always been there for me when I felt a book 'coming on'! Their highly focused proof reading has saved me yet again from numerous errors and has enabled me to send to the printers a text that expresses my ideas clearly, and, please note, who bear no responsibility for any remaining mistakes.

The ideas contained in this publication, however, are my own and are not necessarily shared by any of the institutions for which, or within which, I work.

I have been privileged that this book is the first in ED4MEDPRAC's new publishing enterprise *Aneumi Publications*, and I hope that it will be the forerunner of a range of resources and ideas that will be of use for, and provide support to, all those involved in the complex and important practice of Postgraduate Medical Education.

Della Fish
May 2012

NOTE: There are two authors (Professor David Carr and Professor Wilf Carr) with similar publication dates and broadly similar subject matter, from whom I quote and whose ideas I acknowledge. The need to distinguish them clearly has, of necessity, made some referencing within the text slightly awkward.

I am of course grateful to both writers, but particularly to Professor David Carr within whose many publications about education as a practice I have found much philosophical enlightenment, articulated with enviable precision and vividness about matters that are as important for doctors who are teachers as for those whose profession is teaching. DF

Foreword

This book is for the individual practising doctor and surgeon and all those interested in Postgraduate Medical Education (PGME) and its ramifications for the quality of patient care. This is an important aspect of professional practice which has not received the full attention it deserves within the medical community despite the demand, over many years, for evidence based practice and the more recent requirements to increase the quality of care but to balance this against increased productivity and efficiency. PGME is more than the "traditional" apprentice model of learning with its current traditional focus on motor development, information recall, process management and compliance.

Postgraduate Medical Education involves, in addition to an awareness of one's own knowledge, an understanding of the means of conveying that knowledge in a meaningful way to the learner. This involves contextualising practice, being current and being able to offer knowledge at the depth and level of understanding of the learner. Education is an integrative practice, requiring self-awareness, preparation of the environment (the where and when of learning) and the establishment and maintenance of both one's own knowledge base and that of the learner(s). Education is therefore far more complicated than simply engaging in the superficial "teaching" session. For example how can the teacher discover the existing knowledge base of those to be taught? How will new knowledge be acquired by the learner, in what appropriate order should new knowledge be met, and how will it build on the base of previous knowledge? Further, how does the teacher differentiate between the *theory* of practice and the *habits of custom and practice*?

It has always been acknowledged that the contemporary senior clinician is a valuable repository of knowledge but less recognition is given to their abilities in managing its access by others. Yet the evidence is clear regarding the most effective access routes for learners — for instance: engaging with teachers who are passionate about their subjects; working with clinicians who understand the curriculum and how this guides learning; and using sound assessments to crystallize the quality of progress.

The experience and knowledge of teachers in PGME comes with responsibility both to sustain and enhance care and to develop to the full their fellow clinicians. The public look to those already demonstrating highly proficient clinical abilities also to develop the next generation of practitioners by supporting them on their journey towards their highest aspiration. Reflection is key to this process. Part of this responsibility includes being willing and able to reflect on one's *own* practice. It follows that it requires teachers as educationists who can enhance learning and enable practitioners to contextualise their work such that they provide quality care within the developing movement to regulate postgraduate medical education. Certainly, to focus only on the technical aspects of practice without a moral context removes the responsibility for compassion which enables medical and surgical interventions to enhance the wellbeing of the patient.

This book explores such themes and convincingly argues that Postgraduate Medical Education should be refocused within the moral mode of practice. It addresses the role of the consultants and other clinicians who actually teach in the clinical setting, discusses the principles of learning and assessment in the clinical environment and explores how doctors can enhance their existing educational practice even at the same time as they develop their own clinical expertise.

The argument in this book of why education is a moral practice and its demonstrations of how to engage with this, *in practice,* will rouse the reader to question the current framework for PGME and, it is to be hoped, recognize and develop its potential for future improvement.

Professor Michael Thomas PhD, MA (Law), BSc, RMN, RNT, Cert Ed, FBPS, FHEA
Pro-Vice Chancellor
University of Chester
May 2012

Introduction

Introduction

Starting with a challenge
The impact of the current context on medical educational practice
The argument of this book
The aims of this book
The structure of the book
The readership
The title

Starting with a challenge

This book issues a serious challenge to Postgraduate Medical Education (PGME) in the second decade of the twenty-first century, to look forward *now* to a time when the education of practising doctors within the disciplines of postgraduate medicine and surgery will become a specialty in its own right. It also calls for the re-instatement and further development of a more balanced approach to the education of postgraduate doctors, as was previously enshrined in the *best* practices found in medical and surgical 'firms', before the days of Modernising Medical Careers (MMC). In such firms, 'learning doctors' worked on longer-term and more focused placements with a cohesive group of specialist doctors. They were actively nurtured educationally within these firms (albeit tacitly rather than explicitly) as a person and a professional with developing beliefs, assumptions and values as well as knowledge and skills. They were not simply trained to become a repository of medical facts and a performer of 'mastered' medical procedures. Since MMC, it appears that providing an educational upbringing has become less of a focus for PGME, and been replaced by a very considerable emphasis on training in the technical aspects of medical practice. This book illustrates how that balance could, and should, be redressed.

Arguably, had the medical profession been equipped with a properly principled understanding of the nature of education and of educational thinking — as appropriate to postgraduate medicine — it would not have allowed current PGME to focus only on training. It therefore seems important, before all sight is finally lost of the need for a broader and deeper education of young practising doctors, that there should be an in-depth debate about the roles of education and training within PGME, and about what each might contribute to better patient care.

In order to secure this, and to gain the full understanding, support and involvement of a variety of audiences (from patients, and local managers, to Deaneries and the public), all involved in PGME will need to become rather more expert at explaining clearly its *raison d'être*, educational purposes and rationale, its theoretical bases, and its processes. Engaging in national debate about these ideas, would perhaps also challenge many clinical supervisors' current attitudes to educational activities, where education is still all too frequently seen as training that occurs as an add-on element to be offered only in the space and time round the edge of serious clinical practice.

The impact of the current context on medical educational practice

Evidence has recently begun to emerge, in respect of the state of medical practice and healthcare more generally in Britain in the twenty-first century, of an upsurge in championing the significance of the human spirit and human qualities both in our culture more broadly and in the National Health Service (NHS) in particular. The authors of an important book entitled: *Intelligent Kindness: reforming the culture of healthcare,* 'foreground human qualities rather than competencies, in the delivery of care', in opposition to the dehumanizing influence of the current ethos of our society which values the technical, the instrumental, and the commercial and industrial, and believes in the 'myth of the perfect regulatory system', (Ballatt and Campling, 2011: v - vi). The voice of these authors is only the latest to be raised in opposition to the current culture in healthcare. See also, for example, Iliffe (2008); Neuberger (2006); O'Neill (2002); Pollock (2004); Seddon (2008); and Seldon (2009).

Ballatt and Campling oppose the best natural human qualities like kinship, kindness, attentiveness, attunement and trust, to the unacceptable commodification endemic within concern about targets, numbers, standards, protocols, specifications and bureaucracy. Some of the results of emphasizing such commodification are, they note: coercion, suspicion, anxiety, disempowerment and fragmentation. (Ballatt and Campling, 2011: 173). They call for valuing kindness and the qualities and attributes that characterize it, and add that: 'the culture of education and training would benefit from a consideration of these aims', (*Ibid:* 63). Their book however, is not concerned in detail with medical education as such.

I developed views similar to Ballatt's and Campling's, while working in clinical practice as an educator of postgraduate doctors, and came to a view that, currently in producing doctors who are expert technicians (as required by MMC), we have lost sight of the moral mode of practice, inside which all doctors ought to work (and which patients undoubtedly expect to meet in their medical practitioner). Thus evolved my interest in reshaping PGME in order to develop the kinds of doctors required if medical practice is not — very soon — to lose sight of the importance of the doctor's human qualities.

In offering its ideas, this book takes full account of the importance of the current difficult economic, social and political context of medical practice in relation to teaching postgraduate doctors, but views many of the resulting problems as wrongly construed, and as not at all the most significant issue that PGME currently faces. For example, teaching doctors in the clinical setting is seen as fraught with problems as a result of the European Working Time Directive (EWTD), the requirements of MMC, and the debacle of the Medical Trainee Application System (MTAS), together with the current economic stringencies, as well as the social and media rejection of the status and power of professionals. Thus complaints such as the following arise.

▶ Contact time between learning doctors and their teachers has been reduced recently, so that there is little time for education and thus only the minimum can be achieved.

▷ Doctors are guilty of many errors and their poor training is to blame. This means that they need more training, for which there is no time.

▷ The assessment of doctors in the clinical setting (because it has been narrowly and poorly conceived), has become a bore and a drudge, to be carried out hastily and ticked off speedily, in order not to take time away from real clinical work.

Careful thought will show that these examples (and many like them, that relate to both medical and educational practice) are all conceived of as *technical* problems in search of narrowly technical 'quick-fix' solutions. This, arguably, is what reveals quite startlingly the deeper problem here — that both medicine and education have been re-packaged by MMC as purely technical practices in which we have lost sight of the creativity, sensitivity, flexibility and courage to produce personal rather than protocol-driven decisions and solutions, which professional practices will always require. In short, both the public and practitioners appear to have lost sight of the fact that professional practices like medicine and education require professionals to operate in both the moral as well as the technical mode of practice, where there are moral imperatives to find innovative and more broadly insightful solutions to technical problems.

Indeed, professions have become so rigidly bound by regulation and the threat of litigation that many members have adopted a learnt helplessness in the face of 'the rules', expect to look outside themselves in order to be told what to do, and then accept and thus bow to the conditions that apparently make the problem insoluble beyond a little technical tinkering round the edges. Thus we all forget that the whole point of being a professional is that there are serious responsibilities to take on some agency of our own in shaping our practice, and that a doctor's judgement about a way forward in a context-specific instance may well mean that they need to go beyond the surface and the protocol. Indeed, it may mean going back to first principles and interrogating the taken-for-granted, so as to see things anew.

On this argument, teachers of postgraduate doctors would need to recognize and respond to educational problems as potentially moral as well as technical. They would also need to be more aware of the possibilities for being imaginative in the face of political and other constraints on the education of young doctors. This would mean understanding the wide range of possible educational choices (approaches to teaching, learning and assessment) and selecting these according to the individual context of their learner's need, rather than being content to 'perform' the minimal role currently required of them. Further, they would also need to recognize the vital importance of the serious education of doctors for the future of the profession itself, and then they would protect it as vigorously as they protect their clinical territory. To support this, medical education would need to be seated in a much broader conception of the nature of professional practice and teachers would need to be supported in gaining a much deeper understanding of educational principles. As argued in Fish and Brigley (2010):

> The most crucial point here is that understanding the nature of any practice is an open capacity, not something that can ever be totally mastered. Beginning is the important step. Preparation

can involve reading ... or seeking out a day workshop that offers educational thinking processes. Investigating a small piece of one's own teaching (see de Cossart and Fish, 2005) is another approach. Attempting to set out one's educational values and beliefs is another (but this usually needs professional help from those who are experienced).

(Fish and Brigley 2010: 121)

We also argued for the power of coming together to learn and develop these ideas more extensively with like-minded colleagues, and this can be even more effective if seated within one institution, (see Thomé 2012).

The argument of this book

Thus this book argues that we need to work towards a broadly agreed philosophy about the purposes of and possibilities for postgraduate medical education. It is suggested that this should contain well-thought-through purposes that can be demonstrated to be educationally worthwhile and that are underpinned by a sound and broadly agreed understanding of the nature of educational practice and its processes and choices. This, it argues, is what will enable teachers to be more educationally confident and creative and thus improve the learning of young doctors in the clinical setting, both in terms of what they learn and how they learn it.

Whether we recognize it explicitly or not, the practices of both medicine and education are demonstrably moral enterprises at heart. As will become clear to readers, there are strong arguments for the view that only by espousing a moral as well as a technical view of the nature of practice (both medical and educational) will PGME teachers serve the whole needs of junior doctors and enable them to engage in quality patient care.

The improved educational understanding that springs from exploring these ideas is shown as making for more effective and valuable teaching and learning. It will enable teachers to recognize the importance of the technical skills and knowledge that a practising professional needs to call upon. But it will also attend to the personal character, qualities and values that the doctor ought to bring to meet their patients, and which the teacher should model in their relationship with learners.

Indeed, with hindsight, we can now perhaps see that MMC rightly placed the *technical* education of doctors (the systematic development of vital skills and knowledge) more centrally in clinical practice, and made it more sharply focused on real patient care, supported and supervised by a wider range of clinicians. But it did so to the neglect of (or by making unfounded assumptions about the continuance of) teaching that focused on the moral aspects of practice, as previously provided in the best 'firms'.

In such firms, young doctors stayed long enough to develop, over time, the character, values, and personal qualities constituent of *being a doctor*. In this they were nurtured by a collegiate group of more experienced doctors using the subtle and probably tacit, but no less educational, means of developing in them important habits, modelling for them good professional conduct and engaging them in discussions about practice which raised important questions about what is best for whom and what is the appropriate professional response in given circumstances. As Carr, D. argues: 'good teaching involves the cultivation of positive *personal* relationships' with learners — within, of course, professionally defined rules and principles, see Carr (2005a; 2006). This is important in PGME because what is being developed as doctors practise, is their personal character and judgement, which spring from their personal and professional values, and such development needs the cultivation and nurturing of wiser senior colleagues. This is necessary because a doctor is a moral agent for the patient (making difficult decisions in particular cases for a vulnerable human being) and thus needs to become 'the sort of person or character' capable of putting others first and of making wise judgements about their treatment, since this is what moral agency is all about. Clearly, there are also key parallels for the teacher (see Carr, D. 2007).

Firms, we know, were not all good, but it is arguable that in abolishing them, replacing them by shorter placements, and failing to attend to the longer-term nurturing and developing of those vital personal and professional qualities, MMC has jeopardized the quality of current postgraduate medical education. Further, its intervention (useful as it may have been in some ways) has meant that education in the moral mode of practice is no longer explicitly recognized as a legitimate teaching activity, since nowhere within the current medical and surgical curricula does it feature substantially either in relation to content to be learned or assessment processes to be undertaken.

Fortunately at the moment, the education of doctors in clinical practice is still attended to by many teachers who, as juniors themselves, experienced the development of their own character and conduct. But one wonders what will happen when the new generation of teachers, who did not have that advantage, is left as the almost exclusively educational influence on future doctors' moral awareness!

The aims of this book

The ultimate and longer-term aim of this book, is that *education* for postgraduate doctors, in the moral mode of practice, should become a *recognized practice* in its own right, fully acknowledged as central to the quality of patient care, and researched and developed through *educationally-appropriate* means which have been informed by educationally-driven understanding. This would be in contrast to ill-treating the practice of medical education by acting as if it is intelligible almost exclusively through positivistic research where only that which can be reduced to the measurable is regarded as important.

This requires a wide-ranging debate about what makes for quality in PGME. My immediate aim therefore, is to fuel that debate by *illustrating in depth* how working in the moral mode of practice can provide PGME with a coherent educational philosophy, grounded in real educational understanding that can turn teaching, learning and assessment for practising doctors into something more educationally worthwhile than is generally found at present.

The structure of the book

These aims have, in the first part of this book, resulted in an attempt to explore and reflect upon the nature of professional practice itself (both medical and educational) and to look in new ways at some of the most centrally constitutive elements of teaching and learning as educational activities. This section seeks to stand back and see PGME anew, from an educational viewpoint, and then critique what has previously been taken for granted about it. This leads to a reconsideration of the responsibilities of the medical teacher in PGME, the nature of learning, the relationship of educational theory to practice, the significance of educational aims, and the role of assessment in learning.

The second part of the book then explores the implications of what this reveals for the practice of teaching postgraduate doctors in the clinical setting. It looks in detail at the practical implications for teaching, learning and assessing practising doctors. It offers new approaches to empowering the teacher to make wise educational choices and plan well for coherent teaching in the clinical setting. It considers new ways of thinking about learners and the processes of learning. It shows how to turn informal and formal assessment into a far more educational activity that helps the teacher understand the learner better. And finally, it shows that the quality of PGME should be more about its integrity and identity as a practice engaged in by wise teachers than about its numerical scores on evaluation questionnaires!

Suggestions are made for further reading at the end of every chapter in Part One, starred items being the most highly recommended.

The readership

This book is addressed to all those who seek to understand in some depth what is actually involved in the practices of teaching and learning for practising doctors and surgeons, and how this relates to the quality of patient care. It is targeted particularly at those who seek to develop educationally worthwhile teaching in the clinical setting (clinical and educational supervisors and all who teach doctors in their practice environment). But it also speaks to three other groups. It addresses firstly those who seek to support such teaching in its immediate context (patients and managers). Secondly, it speaks to those who are seeking to develop national standards and systems to regulate — and perhaps also to emancipate — medical education on the ground. This includes all members of the General Medical Council (GMC), Medical Education England (MEE) and its successor Healthcare Education England (HEE), and members and fellows of The Academy of Medical Educators (AoME). Thirdly, and beyond these, it reaches out to those engaged in, or who promote or who read, research in postgraduate medical education.

To gain from this book, readers will require no previous knowledge or experience of 'thinking like an educator' or thinking about education. It offers a critique of the basic current requirements of training courses and why they are inappropriate, and an understanding of why 'tips for teachers', as designed to equip senior clinicians with some basic teaching skills, is a fundamentally inadequate concept. Sadly, examples of this still abound in the recent literature for PGME. Such books offer the false hope that teaching can be improved by cosmetic means, that doctors who teach don't really need much educational expertise and that it is acceptable to squeeze education into as little time as possible. See for example: Dent and Harden (2009); Dobson, Dobson and Bromley (2011); and Jackson, Jamieson and Khan (2007). Some of their ideas are no doubt offered in the interests of saving the time and energy of clinicians exclusively for the all-important hands-on requirements of patient care. But this overlooks the inescapable point that the sound education of doctors is arguably central to good patient care, both now and in the future.

The title

The title chosen for this book indicates an attempt to refocus the emphasis of PGME from training to the *education* of doctors within the clinical setting. It also challenges teachers and learners to make time for education and use that time more profitably. The need for such refocusing arises arguably, because currently junior doctors are undernourished intellectually, educationally and even clinically by being taught almost exclusively within the technical mode of practice where only knowledge and skills are of interest, and where there is little or no development of them as people.

Such refocusing identifies the need to reconceive the aims and nature of PGME in *educational* terms rather than seeing only training as important. The educational understanding needed for this, uses, *but does not rest solely upon*, the study of a wide range of educational theory. Rather, it depends primarily on the teacher's recognition and fulfillment of their moral as well as their technical responsibilities to learners. This, in turn, is grounded in each teacher's understanding of themselves *as an educator,* which can only be achieved by a teacher who has explored their own educational values, who has focused more on acquiring educational capacities and wisdom than on learning to apply formal repertoires of teaching skills and strategies, who has sound knowledge of educational principles and of practical reasoning, and who knows how to study and attend to each individual learner as a person and a professional. This, it is argued, will enable teaching in PGME to be characterized by flexibility, adaptability and courage, and to be based on an understanding of education *as a practice.* This requires preparation to teach that is: intellectually provocative; personally and professionally liberating; that places the learner as central; and that sees assessment as supporting education, not driving it.

This book is intended to be an educational resource for working in the moral mode of *educational* practice, and illustrates what is involved in this. It can be used in parallel with Fish and de Cossart (2007), whose focus is on enabling learning doctors to work in the moral mode of *clinical* practice. Further books in this series will also seek to illuminate this new approach and support medical teachers to engage with it.

Part One

Putting the *education* back into postgraduate medicine:

towards a coherent philosophy

Chapter One

Seeing postgraduate medical education anew: revealing the need for enhanced teaching

The following are typical comments from consultants in discussion with an experienced teacher educator about the very first serious observation of their teaching in the clinical setting.

"I like to think that I encourage people to learn, but when I look at this written account of what happened, I can see that it was not how I thought it was..."

"Planning? Well, my planning is just selecting an example to discuss with a trainee and then helping him or her to look at it in detail."

"I tend to lead the trainee by offering pointers, but not to give them the diagnosis... but if they struggle, it is difficult to know what to do apart from telling them".

Introduction
Starting points: the initial details of the investigation
An analysis and interpretation of the evidence
Absent themes
From the traditional to the enhanced approach to teaching
Enhanced teaching and better patient care
Starting on the journey
Further reading

Introduction

This book is informed by considerable experience over many years of working in clinical practice with senior doctors, whom I observed and advised on their teaching of their juniors. It seeks to begin at a point which many if not most readers will identify as 'where they are' in regard to thinking seriously about education. This will then act as the basis from which to develop more educational understanding, which I believe will in turn lead to the improvement of the practice of teaching, (particularly teaching in the clinical setting), both in postgraduate medical education generally and also for individual teachers.

This chapter demonstrates graphically the need for most doctors to improve and enhance their practical teaching, and briefly sketches what that might involve. The first section describes a modest investigation carried out in 2010 which, though small scale, has produced evidence that also resonates with a far wider range of clinical supervisors and characterizes as fairly typical their approaches to teaching in the clinical setting. Interpretation and analysis of the emerging evidence as presented shows that, though these were all volunteers with an interest in learning more about teaching, none was able to articulate a coherent view of either what educational practice more generally should be about, or of what they were actually attempting in their own teaching. Particularly striking was the absence of understanding about a whole range of basic educational principles.

The chapter then ends by exploring what, by contrast, might characterize an enhanced form of teaching in a similar context. In so doing, it paves the way for chapter two which illustrates what the journey to enhanced educational understanding actually involves and is about, and which illustrates the Aristotelian philosophy that underpins these ideas. This then acts as a platform for the rest of Part One of this book.

Starting points: the initial details of the investigation

The small-scale enquiry conducted in a secondary care setting involved myself, as an experienced teacher-educator and researcher, observing twelve senior clinicians, all in one hospital, each teaching a junior doctor in the clinical setting. Each clinician had secured a place on a Postgraduate Certificate (PG Cert) course, entitled 'Education for Postgraduate Medical Practice', which was validated by Chester University and taught within their own hospital. (See Thomé 2012 for a full evaluation.) The investigation focused on the first of three separate observed sessions for each candidate. This first session occurred just before they began their course, and the other two ran through the first two terms. The group consisted of nine consultants across six specialties; one associate specialist; one specialty doctor; and a very senior nurse who was responsible for skills training throughout medicine within the Trust. (A key requirement to join the course was involvement in teaching postgraduate doctors.) Two of the group had been on a previous PG Cert, and one had attended a Further Education vocational course for teachers. All three claimed that they could remember little about what they had learnt. All twelve had at some point in their careers already completed what was currently the basic and only mandatory support for teachers — that is, some kind of Training the Trainers course. In the event, one of the twelve succumbed to a serious health problem just before the course began and only eleven proceeded — all of them successfully.

The purpose of the investigation was to establish the potential course members' starting points in respect of their educational understanding and their practical teaching. All had volunteered to join the course because of their interest in improving their teaching, but it had become clear at interview that they applied because they were unsure of whether what they had been doing for years was 'right'! In fact 21 had applied and those selected at interview were admitted not only on simple technical criteria of availability and understanding of the demands of the course, but also in the light of flexibility of mind about educational matters.

The first observations revealed a number of common patterns that, it seems reasonable to claim, captured something of the essence of current medical education as offered in the clinical setting in secondary care, by teachers who have mostly had little preparation for their roles as teachers, but who at least were interested in seeking to check out and possibly improve their practice. This state of affairs, in which enthusiastic supervisors of postgraduate doctors are unsure of what teaching involves, is probably still the case for many of the consultants and registrars in our hospitals, although this may be somewhat less true of primary care. And if that is how those who are enthusiastic teachers think, we may be right to worry about those who give less thought to teaching. This small investigation, and the experience that it is more widely representative of, has influenced where this book begins and its view of at least some readers' starting points.

The processes of the investigation

The clinicians being observed for the first time were asked to choose an appropriate learning doctor and an appropriate topic and setting, as close to the norm of their ordinary teaching as possible. All seemed to find this reasonably achievable. What they did and said during their teaching was observed by myself — for all twelve — and was recorded in writing in duplicate at the time (and with timings noted in the margin). One copy was immediately provided for the observed teacher. This then became the direct evidence (read together and analyzed and interpreted on the spot by each of us), for the basis of an hour's private discussion (a professional conversation, not a 'feedback session') between the teacher and myself. This discussion followed the teaching immediately, and set out to probe and explore their aims, their preparation for the session, what they were thinking during the process and their decision-making before and within the teaching. The intention of this entire process was not to engage in any kind of judgemental assessment but rather to provide the basis for an hour's reflective conversation with the teaching doctor about educational and teaching issues that were relevant to that teaching session as observed in that context. On the following day, I privately provided for each teacher my individual written response to their whole session. Again this was not judgemental about structure or process, but was aimed at leading into their course by raising interest in important and relevant educational issues arising from their own practice.

Because this was not a 'formal assessment' process, and because I do not construe teaching as well represented by a de-contextualized list of skills and strategies, there was no 'tick list' for the observation. As will emerge during the book, such 'atomizing' of teaching under headings is only one way of thinking about an educational enterprise, and it was not the preferred one here. Neither did I seek to make the 'traditional noises' (as advised in Training the Trainers and other similar training courses) about what went well and what went badly during the approximately forty-minute session watched. I simply recorded what happened, although of course even the recording was an interpretation at one level, and this fact was itself part of the conversation. In all cases, looking at the written record of their teaching as observed, was highly instructive, because what they *thought* they did during their teaching and how it was responded to, and what they were *actually recorded as doing and receiving in response*, diverged surprisingly (for them).

The following captures the main issues that emerged, from my point of view as an educator, from these observations across all the twelve clinical teachers. As my *interpretations* of what I saw and heard and of what emerged from our subsequent discussion about this, they are, clearly, shaped by my own educational values and by many years of working first in teacher education and then in postgraduate medical education. The emerging themes from this analysis and interpretation, as recorded below, were shared with the whole group and discussed further during the early parts of the course. The whole group made it clear that it offered a fair representation of 'where they were' before the course began — and, as they said emphatically — not only of where they were, but also where many of their colleagues are! Further, this group's recognition of their starting points resonates well with the many professional conversations I have had with several hundred senior doctors in secondary care, across three Deaneries during the last twelve years, all of whom I have had the privilege to observe teaching in the clinical setting, and about a third of whom I have also taught in the classroom.

An analysis and interpretation of the evidence

Only two of the twelve offered any well-thought-out educational aims for their session and no one conveyed clearly to their learners what they were really trying to achieve in the session. Both teachers and learners made many assumptions about the purpose of the session, but few of these were in fact jointly held. Thus, the 'rules of the game' for the session were not clarified (the learner not always seeing the point of what the teacher was doing), nor were the teacher's expectations of them as learners made clear.

None of the observed clinicians had recognized the important balance between having a well-oiled session with very familiar content, and also being open to the ideas, thoughts and experiences of that individual learner, on that occasion. The balance, between teacher keeping to their agenda and recognizing and attending to the learner's emerging agenda, was never overtly considered. Indeed, in keeping to their own agenda, the teachers relieved themselves of much of the burden of using educational professional judgement during their session, but also deprived their learners of personalized learning in which their creative and critical thinking could be exercised. Needless to say, this also diluted the quality of the relationship between teacher and learner, which is the all-important basis of sound education.

I likened this to setting out on a journey with no clear idea of what you are going to do, where you are trying to get to, and how you are going to get there. This is not so much about making detailed written preparation for a teaching session as about having a clear and educational purpose in mind — preferably that relates closely to the needs and interests of that learner, whom the teacher knows as a person. But this does require some sound educational understanding of the choices a teacher needs to make for every teaching session, and how to make them!

An analysis of the group as a whole showed the further following points.

1. All were focused *exclusively* on a specific clinical disease or a particular procedural matter, so that whilst the needs of the patient were fully considered, little account was taken of the wider needs of the learning doctor.

2. Ten out of twelve teachers did seat their teaching directly in the clinical setting (with all its complexities), but the clinical context in which the teaching happened was, in most cases, by no means fully exploited educationally, and thus a vital resource was squandered.

3. The patient's role in the session (where there was a patient present) was not well thought-through. The possible *range* of learning resources offered when a patient was present were overlooked in favour of the traditional and well-tried ones (patient examination and history taking).

4. Where the teaching was about specific cases, no teacher went beyond a basic differential diagnosis, focusing on history taking, clinical examination and test results, but not considering in any detail how to tailor these to the individual patient's needs.

5. Where the teaching was about procedures it was about *how* to do a procedure, rather than including a range of wider educational perspectives.

6. It was not clear how the teacher conceived of the learner's role in the session, indeed many gave their learner no role other than listening.

7. Many of the observed sessions seem to have equated teaching with simply 'presenting information'.

8. There were no expectations that these 'listening learners' might need to write anything down during the session (all behaved as if they would have automatic recall of the whole 40 minutes of the teacher's wisdom). Indeed, only one learner had a pencil and paper with them in the teaching session.

9. Getting the learner to reflect rigorously on their clinical experience was not attended to by anyone, and this was not helped by the fact that little of what happened or was said was captured by either teacher or learner, ready for further consideration.

Indeed, throughout their first observation there was little evidence of their thinking like a teacher and no discussion of how they conceived the *nature* of medical practice itself, let alone how they perceived the *nature* of education and of teaching. Thus the most significant evidence to emerge was the absence, across the whole group, of what education as a practice involves at the level of principle. Serious though this is, it is not surprising, given the paucity of formal help that clinicians across the UK are given about their teaching, even though it is a required element of their posts.

Absent themes

The following list captures the general themes and key educational ideas that were missing across both the first observation and also in the ensuing commentary offered by the observed teacher. When first presented with these, the entire group was clear that such ideas were new to them. The list was discussed at the first session of the PG Cert, again, not in judgemental terms but in order to open up their awareness to a range of matters that teachers need to consider. Many of these became the meat of the first module, and many are explored in detail at the level of principle, in the following chapters. Later in the course, all members of the group were comfortably using and further developing these principles creatively. It will be noted that many points are followed by a question or comment, which was used orally to lead the discussion in class. The whole process was designed to illustrate how teachers think and to show that some aspects of teaching can be enlightened by common sense based on principles and experience!

Frame 1.1   Some important ideas about education not evidenced anywhere during the first observation

1. **Any teaching session should have a discernable structure**, with an educational logic holding the sections together. What structures help you, when you are being taught?

2. **Education should have more coherence than that found in a quick chat in the corridor. The fragmentary nature of learning that seems inevitable because of the nature of service commitments need not be accepted as inevitable.** Teachers need to develop strategies to get round this. Can you think of any?

3. **Highlighting key teaching points as you teach is important.** Teacher needs to have thought through beforehand *for each session* what some of these are, and be on the watch for those that arise in the session. How might you do this?

4. **Teaching is not 'telling' the learner, or 'socking it to them'.** All that is proved when teacher does this, is that teacher knows and understands the topic. How learners make meaning out of it may be much less clear (unless we adopt certain strategies). What might they be?

5. **Teachers need to attend to the needs of learners (who are more important than the teacher).** Teachers need to understand where the learner is, in respect of what they are about to learn, and have a working knowledge of their interests. How can you do this, and when?

6. **Attending simultaneously to several learners who may be at different levels** requires carefully thought-through strategies to ensure a sound educational experience for all involved. Can you think of ways of doing this?

7. **Learners learn best when they are active.** They need things to do, even when your focus and attention is on another learner — also, avoid doing all the talking! A good teacher is a good listener. How do you know whether you are?

8. **Fear of bullying is short-changing your learners.** A number of observed teachers lacked the confidence to challenge their learners to reach beyond their comfort zone. All

learners need a secure and supportive learning environment — *then* you can challenge them and that challenge will not be seen as bullying. Learners need 'stretching' or they will make no progress! How far to challenge a learner to go beyond their comfort zone is the teacher's professional judgement made in that context, on that day, in the light of how the learner is doing. But that doesn't excuse the teacher from having had some thoughts beforehand about where you hope to extend them — and in respect of what — if the opportunity arises.

9. **Getting the *learner* to provide sound and robust evidence** that s/he has developed appropriately or not is important. Ordinary assessment 'tools' in PGME do not do this well, because mostly they record evidence on tick-box forms 'filled in' by teacher! What might a good educator do about this?

10. **Learners need to be helped to develop habits and discipline that will facilitate their learning** (one of these is to require them to have paper and pen ready when they come to you to learn)! What might others be?

11. **Try not to answer your own questions.** Beware of learners who have well-honed strategies for getting you, their teacher, to do their work — for example, getting you to answer your own questions. If this happens frequently, think about the wording of your questions.

12. **Praise too easily earned is un-motivating for the learner, keep it for when it is really deserved.** Find other ways of encouraging! Can you think of any appropriate ones?

13. **Proper and rigourous reflection on practice and experience is vital if the learner is to learn from it. It is reflection on one's experience that reveals its meaning, both in clinical and educational practice.** When do you do this, and when might you do it?

14. **More than facts. There is much more to learn about medicine than the factual medical knowledge and skills.** These are the technical matters with which PGME doctors need you to help them. But there is more than this. 'Being' a doctor is different from knowing like a doctor. What might the difference involve?

15. **Gain more from less. All good teaching and learning that achieves more education in a shorter time has at least 3 sections to it:**
      a) BEFOREHAND the teacher and learner need to prepare appropriately
      b) DURING the session both teacher and learner need to be active and there
      needs to be structure (a discernable beginning, a middle and an end)
      c) AFTER the session the teacher needs to attend in some way to engaging the
      learner in follow-up activities and then to give further response to these.
How does such a structure help the learner?

16. **All teaching sessions need to be contextualized** to what the learner is currently learning from others around you and from what is happening in the clinical setting... it should also relate to what is set out in their curriculum, and the learner's own interests. Do you know the learner's curriculum well?

17. **Simulation.** Some of you taught procedures in a simulated environment for your first observation, and all of you do this from time to time. Some of this is about *'training'*, (following protocols). However, for doctors, there is always more to a procedure than following the protocol. They need to develop good professional judgement, and this (as we shall see) requires *education*. How did you develop yours? Why will it be different now for your learners?

18. **Informal assessments** are an inevitable part of any teaching session! You can't help making *some* rough and ready judgements even as you first meet a learner. These do affect your work with the learner but they may be inaccurate and unfair ... you have to treat them as you would treat intuition, and check out the evidence, before you rely on them! So, what sort of evidence will you seek out — and from where?
Please note that, as we shall see later, informal assessment used educationally is an important means of understanding the learner's current grasp of ideas and practice.

19. **Educational Judgement.** The good teacher is involved in making sound educational judgements that involve knowing the range of options available for a given educational intention and selecting the one that is best for the given learner in a given context. Such decisions often have to be finalized on the spot at the time.... (If that seems familiar, that is because good clinicians do this for patients about the range of clinical options available). How did you learn to make good clinical judgements?

20. **Teaching them to think.** The thinking processes of learning doctors need careful and precise development. This cannot be learnt at medical school because students do not have full responsibility for a patient. The teacher's role therefore is to understand the detail about their own clinical thinking and to make their expert thinking and judgements explicit. Then they can help learners to do the same! At what level of *detail* do you already do this?

These are about the teacher's responsibility to their learner. This is a moral responsibility — unless the teacher is content to offer just the technicalities the learner needs.

For those who have already thought carefully about the nature of education and therefore have established an educational philosophy that drives their practice, these would be very elementary points. But those observed found it hard on that first occasion to envisage any other ways of operating beyond the simple technical approaches of 'telling and asking' their learners and focusing on the simple technical content of medical knowledge and procedures. They were, seemingly, all caught up in the traditional technical approach to teaching and had no view beyond it. This may have been because their teaching had been influenced by the training approach taken by Training the Trainers and other similar training courses.

The following provides the first indications that there is indeed another approach and a different way forward for medical educators.

From the traditional to the enhanced approach to teaching

Behind much of the teaching I have regularly observed on a first occasion in the clinical setting, in secondary care particularly, has lain a very traditional and instrumentalist view of postgraduate medical education, which this book argues is now outmoded, no longer appropriate, and which needs to be superseded by a more educationally informed approach. This impoverished view sees teaching as aimed at 'equipping the workforce to do the job', by simply presenting to, or providing learners with, training in the required knowledge, specific job-skills and procedural methods, as required in current practice. This uninspiring vision, which has more of training for commerce and trade about it than of the development of professional practice, is liable in the context of PGME to produce bored learners — and teachers. It also brings with it a false assumption that assessment is a means of controlling learners and ensuring that they have jumped through sufficient hoops in respect of what they must learn, in order to be 'safe workers' and thus allowed to progress through their careers. This is a highly dubious assumption when related to *patient safety*. To see assessment as a self-standing chore requiring the completion of as many forms as possible, as fast as possible — irrespective of their educational quality — is to make the common mistake of assuming that more is necessarily always better!

What is lacking in these instrumentalist ideas is that they have not been based in a thought-through educational philosophy appropriate for the education of professionals. Further, they cannot contribute to improved patient care because they draw upon, and focus the learning doctor down onto, tried and tired examples which simply replicate the teacher's current clinical practice, and do not allow learners to see beyond the immediate, to challenge the orthodox, to critique the processes, and to recognize the human being behind the façade of the patient.

In writing about this a colleague and I suggested that the instrumental view of teaching:

> often produces teachers with a narrow mindset about education and professional practice, and also provides clinical [and educational] supervisors with little support for the professional practice of teaching. For example, it leaves them to use whatever teaching technique comes to mind (rather than equipping them to make an informed choice from the gamut of educational possibilities), or to copy what was done by those who taught them (without critiquing that approach), or to deploy some off-the-peg tips and tactics derived from "training the trainers" or the "adult learning" movement (without the means of assessing whether the formula these provide is appropriate in the particular case).
>
> *(Fish and Brigley 2010: 113)*

We further argued that traditional clinical teachers often lack an internalised educational structure to facilitate the learner's development, systematically and rigorously and with coherence and progression. We added that the teaching typical of this instrumentalist approach:

> frequently leads to inaction, boredom and disengagement for learners because it only partially engages them. Particularly, it does not attend to developing the intellectual and critical, creative and imaginative abilities of those in whose hands the future development of their profession lies. Also it fails to respond with sophistication to the increasing complexity and uncertainty of the learning context and does not support learners in ways that encourage aspiration to a high level of achievement for themselves and their professions.
>
> *(Fish and Brigley 2010: 113-14.)*

Such a traditional approach to teaching has been inculcated in mentors and supervisors (deliberately or by default) through many *training* programmes. Sadly it has obscured for many clinical teachers the possibility of aspiring to something better, so that relatively few in PGME have ever had the opportunity to be initiated into the traditions of teaching and the subtleties of education as a practice.

By contrast to the instrumental view, we proposed a form of 'enhanced' teaching which would rest 'on a deeper understanding of the nature of education as *emancipatory*' (for the learner and the teacher). We also saw the practice of teaching as 'enabling learners to become more critical, creative and thoughtful practitioners'. We dubbed it 'enhanced teaching' and defined it within PGME as: 'teaching that is based upon in-depth educational understanding, which, in turn, arises from teachers' exploration of and reflection on their own clinical and educational values' in relation to real practice. We also saw this as attending to and seeking to develop learners' understanding and values. (See Fish and Brigley 2010: 114.)

Further, traditional instrumental approaches to teaching (as still offered in PGME courses and textbooks) seem to make little impact on the quality of patient care because such approaches do not treat the learning doctor *as a person*, and are often not even remembered in any detail subsequently. By contrast enhanced teaching achieves considerably more.

Enhanced teaching and better patient care

Most crucially, we argued that enhanced teaching provides a better way of improving the quality of learning in clinical practice, and therefore is a much sounder way of protecting patient safety and fulfilling the demands of clinical governance. This is because it attends directly to the individual doctor as a person and to their practical clinical responsibilities in terms of ethics and values, as well as to their clinical skills and knowledge in relation to the individual patient. In short it equips them to meet the patient and to bring to their care a reservoir of human as well as a technical resources.

The following table (*Table 1.1 Towards a shared purpose in PGME for better patient care*), indicates what this can mean in practice, and is taken from ideas I developed for a major project designed to introduce enhanced teaching into a hospital Trust. The project's intention was to develop within several areas of one Trust a shared understanding between senior and local managers on the one hand and teaching clinicians on the other, about how better educational purposes and processes can directly improve patient care, and thus to agree to facilitate the time and space required for this improvement. This is because many managers do not know what goes on in the name of 'teaching' in medical education (or fear that it is indeed boring, time-consuming and irrelevant to patients), and thus do not begin to understand its crucial role in safeguarding patient safety and improving patient care. As a result they are often understandably disinclined to support educational ventures. The table however, helps to demonstrate the value to patient care of enhanced teaching approaches, and contrasts these with the current instrumental provision, and it indicates why time and space are needed to put this in place in the *clinical setting*.

Table 1.1 Towards a shared purpose in PGME for better patient care

Instrumental approaches involve the following	Enhanced teaching approaches involve the following
Teaching Telling a learner quickly what to do to care for the patient, and then just getting on with the job. This treats the learner as a worker to be instructed. (This is unlikely to impact on improved patient care.)	Engaging *with* a learner in thinking deeply about specific patient care (reflection *in* and *on* action in cases and procedures).
Assessment Teacher completing a traditional national assessment form, without exploring the case with respect to the learner's understanding of the deeper issues raised.	Engaging in a detailed discussion about and assessment of patient care and also the learner completing a record of their clinical insights gained from this process.
Teaching Telling a learner to improve their professionalism.	Seeking to nurture the learner as a doctor who knows who s/he is as a person and a professional (developing, character, disposition and the capacity to know oneself).
Assessment Using the assessment forms to indicate that this needs to be, or has been, attended to.	Reflecting orally and in writing on *professionalism* and *values* in action with patients.
Teaching Telling a learner to *do it my way* — like this.	Helping a learner to adapt the knowledge and skills they have learned in the classroom to safe and caring patient care, across a range of patients.
Assessment Using the assessment forms to indicate they can 'do it as they have been taught to'.	Reflecting orally and in detail on what they have learned through patient cases.
Teaching Telling a learner how relate to patients in a range of contexts (including breaking bad news) — by training them in communication skills.	Supporting a learner as s/he develops their own therapeutic relationship with a wide range of patients.
Assessment Using the assessment forms to indicate this has been attended to.	Reflecting orally and in writing on what they offer in interpersonal relationships with patients and the complexities/problems, the ethical and moral issues and the sensitivities that arise.

What can be seen from this table is that the instrumental approach (on the left), represents what the learning doctor is told to do, which is then assessed simply for whether they can do it *as taught*. This can produce a young doctor who is dependent on their senior as the person who controls their doing, thinking and even 'being' in the clinical setting. This does not readily produce a pro-active, thinking expert on whom any Healthcare Provider can begin to rely to provide best patient care whatever unexpected difficulties occur within treatment. The instrumental approach produces the kind of doctor who is best only at following known pathways and often does not develop the flexibility, creativity and confidence in self that is needed when treating patients who themselves readily discern what their doctor brings to their care. It seems fair to claim that teaching doctors in an instrumental way which equips them only for the expected and predictable, may have led to the unease found currently — amongst doctors, managers and patients — about what junior doctors can actually do!

By contrast to this, enhanced teaching (together with its approach to assessment), as seen in the right hand column, can cultivate a doctor who is learning 'to think' like a doctor' and 'to be' a doctor, in the fullest sense. This is education in its truest sense. A learning doctor under this approach can bring for detailed discussion, exploration, development and refinement with a senior, their own current knowledge and understanding, their own ways of seeing things, and the person they are as a doctor. What they can then offer to patients is a doctor who responds person to person to the patient as an individual with particular health needs, such that almost whatever happens, they can provide for their needs — effectively, efficiently and with the kind of humanity that patients particularly recognize and value when they meet it. This in turn means that the doctor and patient can work together and contribute together towards the best treatment possible. Such a state of affairs is also likely to reduce complaints and to contribute to the Healthcare Provider's reputation for quality care. Further, this may well cost no more, requiring only the reorganization of time and resources. In fact, if the safety and improvement of patient care really matters, Healthcare Providers need to recognize that they cannot afford not to engage with this approach to educating their doctors.

Starting on the journey

In Fish and Brigley 2010: 114, we made the point that we have 'been privileged to see clinicians who, having thought deeply about these matters, have learnt to base their teaching on understanding education as a practice and who have experienced a change of mindset that makes teaching more enjoyable and enhances their learners' experience'. This has recently been further re-enforced by evidence shown in the evaluation of the PG Cert that was based upon the ideas in this book, as carried out by Thomé in 2012.

In Fish and Brigley 2010, we also argued that it is not difficult to begin to understand the nature of education as a practice and that those who are serious can quickly and easily start upon the life-long process of becoming enhanced teachers. Understanding the nature of any practice can never be totally mastered. Beginning the process needs to start with thinking about what is involved in education, and attempting to set out one's educational values and beliefs. We concluded our chapter thus.

Teaching is a professional practice. Members of that community of practice improve by means of critical dialogue and commitment to shared values and ways of working. Ultimately, teacher development involves learning from and with other teachers, face to face (Lieberman and Miller, 2008). Enhanced teachers (and those who seek to become such) will therefore seek actively to engage with the professional and research networks of like-minded colleagues, in whatever ways are practical.

(Fish and Brigley 2010: 121)

Enhanced teaching can never be mastered, being an open capacity, but it is possible to begin on a journey towards it, which is a journey in search of educational wisdom and, as we shall see, expertise in practical reasoning. The next chapter offers a vision of that journey which is really about acquiring educational understanding (of self as a clinician and a teacher, of the nature of medical practice and of the subtleties of educational practice and its use of educational theory). That understanding, it is here argued, will ultimately lead to wiser practice and safer patient care.

Further Reading

Fish, D. and Brigley, S. (2010) 'Exploring the Practice of Education' in J.Higgs, D. Fish, I. Goulter, S. Loftus, J-A. Reid and F.Trede (eds), *Education for Future Practice*. Rotterdam: Sense Publications (chapter 10: 13-122).

Chapter Two

Seeing our aspirations anew: mapping the journey towards educational *praxis*

What those of us need to aspire to who are properly ambitious for our learner's sake to become seriously wise and practically expert teachers, is not so much to acquire extensive knowledge from the various landscapes of educational theory, nor huge repertoires of teaching skills and strategies (however much we may draw on each), but to develop a moral sensibility that shapes how we harness ways of enquiring into the moral and ethical needs of each of our learners — as found in each new teaching context. The question then for educators is how best can we set out to fulfill the expectations that then arise, of us as a teacher, not for fame or fortune sake but rather, only for the sake of doing the best we can.

(Based loosely upon Carr, D. 2000: 102.)

'For us there is only the trying. The rest is not our business.'
T.S. Eliot: Burnt Norton, *Collected poems 1909 – 35*. London: Faber and Faber.

Introduction
The mountain of educational *praxis*: starting on the pathway
An overview of the journey
Aspirations for your journey
Where this way of thinking comes from: what Aristotle can teach us
Further reading

Introduction

The following offers a way of understanding how to work towards providing enhanced teaching in PGME by acquiring the virtue of moral wisdom. This chapter illustrates how this involves climbing beyond the current traditional and instrumentalist approaches to teaching. It also demonstrates what this climb asks of the teacher, since the journey is demanding but rewarding. This is, as will become only fully apparent much later in this book, a journey towards virtue — and ultimately towards virtue for its own sake. For the moment however, starting on the pathway is the most important move any teacher can make who is ambitious to enhance their educational practice and who recognizes the moral imperative to become a better educator — for the sake of learning doctors, their patients, for medical practice and the medical profession, and ultimately for virtue's own sake.

What follows uses an extended metaphor to explain as vividly as possible the vision, the aspirations and the demands associated with refocusing PGME.

The mountain of educational *praxis*: starting on the pathway

Since many doctors and surgeons like to climb mountains (actually or metaphorically), I use this image to illuminate what I am beginning to see as a kind of hierarchy in respect of learning to work with learning doctors — whether physicians or surgeons — as a wise educator. The hierarchy is expressed in *Figure 2.1 The mountain of educational practice*, which needs to be read from the bottom upwards. It shows **training** as occurring separately, on the grassy slopes beneath the educational mountain proper, because it is a different practice from the practice of education, and the role it plays in PGME is somewhat more basic than is the challenge offered within education.

A range of approaches to teaching and learning on the mountain of educational practice can take the aspiring teacher up through the foothills of the climb to about a third of the way to the top. These foothills are the home of **'edu-action'** because here the teacher's activities mimic the actions of education as a practice but without actually being driven by educational understanding.

By contrast, serious expertise in engaging in education as a practice, will take teachers up the final and educational part of the mountain, towards the mountaintop, which is the home of **educational *praxis***. This is about recognizing and understanding the gamut of educational choices available and being able to engage in practical reasoning (just as a doctor engages in clinical reasoning), to choose the best possible educational care for that particular individual's educational needs, as analyzed *in situ* by the teacher and shaped in collaboration with that learner.

Thus, as we shall shortly see in more detail, *praxis* within education, is also about the teacher seeking the best for a learner *for best's own sake* and not, for example, to please a learner, for the cleverness of being a technician or for the fame of being an expert. Further, like reflection, *praxis* can only be truly engaged in from within the moral mode of practice. Indeed, both *praxis* and reflection are inevitably distorted when exercised within the technical mode of practice, because it is inimical to them.

Praxis requires creating wise judgements in response to on-the-spot needs, rather than obeying previously designed technical procedures and protocols to gain personal success. It uses artistic rather than technical means, and uses them to genuinely virtuous and often unforeseen ends. It therefore cannot be taught by providing lists of questions to ask whenever an occasion arises to the end of shaping a learner to a pre-designed technical model of perfect technician. Indeed, *praxis* for a teacher is about 'acquiring capacities to ask ever more complex, sophisticated and evaluative questions about that important aspect of human flourishing called education' (Carr, D. 2000:90).

The details are as follows.

Figure 2.1 An overview of the mountain of educational practice
(to be read from the bottom upwards)

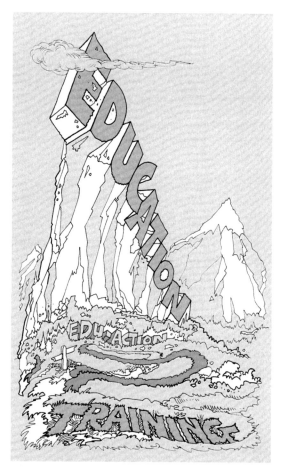

EDUCATION

> **Engaging in educational
> *praxis* as a life-long
> journey**
>
> ↑

**3. Understanding the nature
of *praxis***

> **Engaging in the practice
> of education**
>
> ↑

**2. Understanding the nature of
education and self as a person
and an educator**

> **Engaging in the practice
> of teaching**
>
> ↑

1. Thinking like a teacher

EDU-ACTION

iii. Using *ad hoc* random elements
of theory

ii. Doing what teachers appear to
do

i. Following tips for teachers

TRAINING
Adhering to the requirements of
Training the Trainers

An overview of the journey

As Figure 2.1 shows, the grassy slopes where teachers are content to behave as trainers, lie below the mountain proper, and only beyond this does the mountain of educational practice itself begin to rise. On the lower third of the mountain proper, the teacher seeks to perform more like an educator than a trainer (though without totally understanding what is involved in the complexity of education). On reaching the upper two thirds, the teacher seeking to enhance the education they offer learners can gain the necessary understanding to set them on a truly educational journey that involves development through three stages. The detail is as follows.

The grassy slopes beneath the mountain where training occurs

By means of this metaphor, training is placed on the grassy slopes at the very foot of the mountain proper because it involves drilling learners in new behaviour, but without engaging the learner's thinking processes. This has its uses wherever we wish to inculcate important habits that need to become tacit and automatic in learners to enable them to move to higher levels of intellectual and/or skills-based endeavour. In learning to learn in the clinical setting, for example, new doctors may need to become adept at educational routines and adopt habits that enable them to benefit from teaching offered in a far more complex setting than found in their medical school. And in surgery, for example, certain craft skills have to be learnt through training (known as basic surgical training), where simulation allows practice that cannot compromise patient care. However, training is not the same as education, and is therefore seen as separate from the mountain proper. Training may, for example, enable the practice of technical procedures but it cannot cultivate a surgeon who is aware of the importance of professional judgement and who knows when, where and how to utilize their skills in the healthcare setting and who does so with sensitivity, humanity and where necessary, improvisation.

Training attends to inculcating in the learner routine skills and procedures, so that they become immediate behavioural responses to a commonly occurring stimulus (event). Training is *done* to the trainee, and is done by a teacher who works as an obedient agent of someone else's ideas which in the case of 'Training the Trainers' and other similar training courses, are laid down in a nationally agreed programme. This acts like the nationally available menu provided in pubs belonging to chains, where the fare has been pre-organized so that it can be reproduced in every member-pub on every occasion. Such training enables any supervisor to be prepared as a teacher, in exactly the same way, by anyone who is an accredited trainer for that course. Thus, every course attendee will, by the end, be expected to behave exactly as trained. This may promote 'safe and reliable' routine behaviour, but it does not prepare them for those contexts in which the scenario does not call for formulaic behaviour. It also sees the teacher as promulgating someone else's content and processes. Such teaching cannot, therefore be construed as a moral enterprise, since both trainer and trainee have lent themselves to serve someone else's ends, and the trainee is offered no choice, because they are not invited to think about the means and ends of what they are being trained to do. Rather they are being 'instrumentalised', (see Macklin 2009).

Learning the complexities of being a doctor in clinical practice is unlikely to be well served by extensive training. Whilst learning to perform clinical routines without thinking may at first sight seem important, medicine is full of complexity, particularity and uncertainty and often does not yield to the application of pre-learnt and rigid protocols. Indeed, there is anxiety amongst many doctors that protocols might be as likely to jeopardize patient safety as to ensure it and that in many contexts, guidelines requiring thought may be safer than an absolute formula. For this reason, postgraduate (trainee) doctors' and surgeons' main needs are to develop sound clinical thinking, good decision-making, and wise clinical judgement, based upon deep understanding (which lies beyond knowledge). These they need to learn to use alongside developing a range of personal and professional characteristics and qualities, in the service of particular patients. Only education can fully attend to such matters.

It is surely ironic therefore, that even at the beginning of the second decade of the 21st century, clinical and educational supervisors in PGME are still expected as a minimum by the GMC simply to use attendance at the Training the Trainers course as the preparation for teaching postgraduate doctors. This is especially shocking since these courses, originally designed in the 1990s are only now beginning to be upgraded. It is also unfortunate that this approach continues to be emphasized in the UK, by ubiquitously referring to senior doctors as 'Trainers' and those who learn from them as 'Trainees'. Arguably, what is needed instead at postgraduate level are teachers who offer learning doctors an educational approach. The transition from training to education that safe medical practice requires is thus represented in the mountain metaphor by a change of terrain and angle of the slope encountered as the trainer strives to become an educator. This signals the need for a change of understanding and of mindset with respect to education.

The foothills of the mountain where 'edu-action' occurs

Climbing in the foothills of the mountain represents (for very many) the first stages of such striving. Most clinical supervisors who see training as necessary but not sufficient and who wish to offer trainees something better, inevitably climb on this part of the mountain. They are seekers, but are usually without serious educational support. As a result, they strive alone to find a better approach to teaching, but whilst seeing through the training approach and avowing the need to do better for their learners, they struggle to know what this might actually mean.

The danger on this part of the mountain is that like real climbers the unwary medical teacher can follow paths that mislead or peter out. Thus, whilst seeking to become an educator, because they do not yet really fully understand what education involves, they can be seduced into 'going through the motions of education' but without recognizing that something more intellectual lies beneath the teaching that is educationally worthwhile. That is why this stage of the mountain is labelled 'edu-action'.

Three pathways provide examples of this. All three involve the teacher making changes to their performance, but without realizing that teaching is not only about performance, and that some performances do not even enhance learning. One such strategy on the pathway of edu-action, involves relying on tips for teachers. The second relates to teachers behaving as they remember their own best teacher seemed to do (but without perhaps recognizing that what they saw would only have been the visible aspects of being a teacher)! The third involves, having attended perhaps a one-day course or read an article or chapter on some aspect of educational theory, immediately adopting these ideas and applying them *ad hoc* and uncritically to all practice, as if they constitute *the* ultimate theoretical base (which in fact does not exist).

On the first pathway, **following tips for teachers**, aspiring postgraduate medical educators pick up a few 'educational' tips, which have been put together by someone else who does not know their specific context. These tips are mostly commonsense ideas that have been temptingly summarized for use by everyone. Inspection of these, however, will soon show that they are either so general that they fit every possibility and are thus useless outside totally routine practice, or that they are dangerous, because they can run out when the unexpected happens in practice and leave the teacher stranded with no means of working out what to do next. This is because they do not own the thinking that underpins the tips.

A second pathway offers a strategy called '**doing what my best teachers seemed to do**' (where their own 'good' teachers from the past become the model that shapes behaviour). Here, the medical teacher sets out to mimic the visible aspects of teachers they remember. This again is about adopting someone else's way of working. Further, it is fraught with dangers. Because their own teachers made it look easy, aspiring teachers assume that teaching is no more than the visible aspects of practice — a mere matter of common sense applied at the time and driven by fairly obvious routine ways of doing things. However, not actually *being* the model they mimic, not having the same characteristics, not knowing what underpinned the observed behaviour, and not using these strategies in the same context as their model did, aspiring teachers will find in the end that this approach is no guide to what to do when the model falls short of what is appropriate. Teachers behaving in this way, then, are no more their own agents than those who follow tips for teachers.

Those following a third pathway may appear to have a better chance of getting somewhere useful. They for example **learn some elements of theory** that they have seized upon magpie-like from books or workshops, but which they have chosen *ad hoc* and without any awareness of how they fit into the much wider landscape of educational theory and practice as a whole. Like the rest climbing on the 'edu-action' section of the mountain however, such teachers do not really own the thinking that has informed those theories, and also do not recognize that 'theories' are only someone's ideas and constructs which are only as sound as the thinking behind them and only as useful as each new educational context permits. Further, these teachers do not have a holistic view of teaching. They neither know what role educational theory can safely play in practice, nor how to theorize their own educational practice through reflective enquiry. They too, therefore, have no means of knowing what to do when the 'given theories' run out of use.

Thus, all three sets of climbers in the edu-action foothills of the mountain are influenced by a loosely connected set of *ad hoc* ideas, and are very much someone else's agent in terms of what they teach and how they teach it. Although their teaching is driven by the very best motives, (and such motives are the pre-cursor to finding genuinely better ways forward as sound educators), they are in fact going through the motions of education without understanding its underpinning intellectual bases and without knowing how to think like a teacher. Indeed, it is ironic that in their own profession of medicine, they would never set out to treat a patient without being familiar with and knowing how to use the appropriate theoretical knowledge, without serious experience of thinking like a doctor, and without knowing or being able to work out what the appropriate treatment options were in this individual case. Sound education requires a similar set of abilities.

It should be re-emphasized that this short-fall in understanding is not the fault of those seeking to do better for their learners, because few teachers in PGME have had much formal support of any kind for providing education in general (let alone preparation for offering education for postgraduate professionals). Thus on this part of the mountain, they are likely to be on pathways that will run out on them, and without meaning to, they will at some point inevitably short-change their learners. Their ideas are not their own, because they are not part of a coherent personal educational philosophy that they have worked out. Thus they cannot make educationally wise decisions for themselves or for their learners.

Equipped with an understanding gained from their own experience then, that these lower slopes are inadequate or lead nowhere, those who seriously wish to, or who are convinced of their moral responsibility to become a sound educator, will ultimately find and set out on the pathway that leads upwards and makes more profitable use of their time and energy. For this, they may need a guide or guides who will quickly enable them to see the shortcomings of the foothills and who will then help them place their feet at the start of the higher slopes that lead unfailingly upwards towards educational practice.

The upper slopes of the mountain where the enhanced teacher aspires to educational praxis

Placing one's feet on the first stage of the upper slopes will open up new educational and self-understandings that will inevitably lead to better thinking about teaching and thus improved practice. Further exercise on these slopes will develop on the second stage, enhanced teaching, which becomes genuinely educational practice where the focus is on education which is worthwhile because it contributes to the learner's and the teacher's flourishing. For some, the intellectual and moral lure to seek to become an expert will lead them towards educational *praxis*, a third and final stage that will actually engage them in a life-long journey. Here, a teacher's motivation changes from technical and self-serving ends to the virtuous aspiration of doing one's best — for others and ultimately for its own sake. Here, cultivating the virtues is 'not just a means to a flourishing life, but [is] what a flourishing life *means*' (Carr, D. 2007: 379).

Thus, those reaching these upper and more advanced slopes of the mountain will find themselves working through the first two stages and perhaps towards the third, in order to develop their expertise — which will also equip them to continue to climb to more and more challenging heights. In climbing these more difficult slopes towards the top of the mountain, teachers will recognize the need to develop a coherent understanding of educational thinking. This can be done by both exploring and investigating their own teaching practice reflectively and by enlightening their emerging understanding with deeper study of what is involved both in the practice of education and in what we can safely say about — but also what we should not expect of — its theoretical underpinning. This process, as we shall see, is intrinsically motivating in that such climbing becomes personally as well as professionally interesting and challenging, and where we find that success brings further and also higher aspiration.

The three stages of difficulty for the climbing teacher on this educational part of the mountain are found on slopes the first of which rises upwards from beginning to understand the *process of teaching* (coupled with beginning to engage thoughtfully and reflectively in the practice of teaching). From this then emerges growing understanding of the wider and deeper *process and practice of education* (coupled with beginning to engage in educational practice). Finally at the top of the mountain, climbers begin to experience the life-long journey of developing educational *praxis*.

The first of these three stages, on the upper slopes of the mountain, is about **thinking like a teacher** and beginning to understand the process of teaching. This sees the teacher starting to accrue the knowledge, understanding and confidence to go beyond the efficient 'delivery' of teaching — which is mostly training — to facilitating the learner in acquiring new understanding. Here we see climbers who are beginning to acquire a range of specific skills and strategies that teachers use, and who gradually start to formulate principles for when, where, how and why to use them. Learning as a process also begins to be focused on, and understanding is developed of more sophisticated ways of enabling learners to learn (beyond telling them, instructing them and lecturing to them with predictable PowerPoint presentations). Yet at this first educational level, the aspiring teacher does not yet fully see the learner *as a particular person* and there appears as yet little personal basis for seeing and thinking about teaching (a personal philosophy of teaching). This might be seen as looking at teaching from outside its practice (a theoretical perspective) as opposed to engaging in that practice, which is why this stage needs to be united with **engaging in the practice of teaching.**

The teacher who aspires to improve their practical teaching by engaging thoughtfully in the practice of teaching, will learn to use and develop further their understanding of both themselves as a teacher and their teaching in and during practice. This involves seeing oneself as a professional teacher who makes and implements decisions about how to teach, based on some theoretical understanding about teaching and learning, plus a growing experience of teaching as a practice in its own right. Here, teaching begins to be seen as a more complex process than previously perceived and as being driven by serious responsibilities to learners. In short, the climber begins to think like a teacher, and gradually becomes well-informed about teaching as a practice.

The second stage on these educational slopes involves the aspiring teacher in **beginning to understand the nature of education as a practice — and also to understand themselves better as persons as well as educators.** This means the aspiring medical educator both being aware that education, like medicine, is a values-based practice with a moral heart, and also becoming conscious of the values that drive their own practice in both of these professions. This in turn means recognizing both the contribution to teaching made by their own character and personal philosophy, and seeing teaching as a moral enterprise with major responsibilities. This also means having consolidated the knowing and understanding that make for enhanced teaching. Such teachers, who begin to see themselves as educators, also make and implement thoughtful educational decisions about working with their learners. Here then, teaching (and the preparation for it) begins to be more imaginative (well beyond technical performance and skill), and education is recognized as promoting 'the moral, psychological and physical well-being of learners' (Carr, D. 2000: 9). It should be noted however, that the role of theoretical studies in gaining this stage of understanding educational practice is not perhaps as central as many have suggested in the past. Thus, the 'understanding' discussed above is not pre-eminently formal *theoretical* understanding. Chapter seven explores these ideas in more detail.

Thus, a climber at this level develops, records and keeps under review their own personal educational philosophy or creed and critiques and shares it in order to continue to develop it. Alongside this, they become more the person they are and come to know themselves more deeply — both as educators and doctors! (There is even evidence that this affects their own clinical practice in positive ways, see Thomé 2012.) Thus they become the educator who meets their learner more confidently as a person. In medical education, this is particularly important because doctors are routinely brought up to hold themselves back within their medical practice to a distance that enables them to cope with the difficult demands of life and death, whereas in education, the character and personal qualities of the teacher are quite inextricably bound up within the education they offer to learners.

Equipped with some sense of the complexity of the practice of teaching that is educationally sound, climbers at this stage become ready to grow into **engaging in the practice of education.** In short, they begin to think like an educator and to practise as one. They are drawn to analyze what their learners, as individuals, need and they recognize the difference between what a learner 'wants' and what they 'need'. They conduct themselves like serious educators who see practice as based on deep understanding and professional judgement, and who have an active personal philosophy about education. Educators of this kind gradually begin to act as reliable, principled and well-informed educational agents, who (guided by educational understanding) are able to choose wisely how best to develop the doctors of the future and when to bow to the requirements of other agencies.

Finally, the pinnacle of educational expertise, as illustrated at the top of the mountain, is about **engaging in educational *praxis* as a life-long journey.** This can never be mastered. It is a concept from the philosophy of Aristotle but recurring in works of many key educational thinkers ever since. (For a recent example, see Bondi, Carr, Clark and Clegg 2010.)

Praxis can be seen in a number of guises, some nearer to Aristotle's original vision than others. Essentially it involves engaging in practical reasoning, or deliberation. Indeed, in principle, this process is, at its best, the same as that found in medical practice in respect of treating the patient. *Praxis* means being able to envisage each of the gamut of educational choices available in a given context (in respect of teaching, learning and assessment), choosing the best purpose and the best means to achieving it for this learner, and then being able to use this to engage in educationally worthwhile practice that is the best available educational experience for that learner in their context. Clearly, given evaluative words like 'best' and 'worthwhile', this has a moral thrust to it.

However, the ultimate key to the pinnacle of *praxis* is related to the motivation for engaging in it. Where this is to achieve good technical ends, even *praxis* can be twisted into a technical process. For example, it can be treated as a formulaic way to 'do the best for the learner' in order to be a good teacher. An example might be, in order to shine as a teacher, to ask in each situation where deliberation is needed (in preparation for teaching, during teaching and after it), the following sorts of questions.

▷ What are my immediate educational intentions?

▷ What else will I be / might I be teaching 'inadvertently' or concomitantly?

▷ What in this context should direct my actions?

▷ What more skills do I need to do this well?

▷ What clearer moral vision do I need to act wisely?

▷ What does greater criticality say about what I am *really* doing here? (What are the longer-term results of my teaching as well as the short term ones?)

Such a teacher certainly sees education as a moral and an intellectual endeavour and enjoys the problem-solving nature of deliberating about what is best for the given context and given set of learners in their own practice. Such a teacher is also poised to develop creatively new ideas and understandings both about education (for him-/herself) and also to encourage the creativity of their learners. Their ultimate aim would be to see their learners go beyond them in their achievements and understanding. Doctors and surgeons will recognize the parallels here with the *praxis* of medicine and surgery.

It should be noted, however, that beyond this is a view of *praxis* that sees it as springing from not just a disposition towards natural virtue (being moved, for example, to do good, with perhaps a hope of some recognition for this) but *arising from* genuine virtue (having a disposition to good, and to do good, for its own sake, and a commitment to wisdom). See Carr, D. 2005b: 143; and, Kemmis and Smith (eds) 2008: 15-35. This is about leading the moral life in 'which moral growth is more a matter of the lifelong cultivation of character and capacities for good character-forming judgement' (Carr, D. 2005b: 148). Carr makes the key point here that literature and art are a prime source of moral insight for experiencing 'the consequences for moral flourishing of character and choice', and for having 'a special role to play in the education or refinement of affect'. In this he places poetry above the rest of the arts. Elsewhere (Carr 2000: 90), he suggests that development of new teachers might be better achieved through the arts than through an *over*emphasis on the role of educational theory in our understanding of the nature of education, and that we can 'overestimate the value of theoretical studies in professional education for teaching'.

The minimum requirement for teaching postgraduate doctors

Currently, as this book goes to print, the minimum qualification for teaching postgraduate doctors in the clinical setting is having attended a 'Training the Trainers' course of no more than two or three days duration. This minimum requirement has remained at the same level for many years. Arguably, the quality of teaching in postgraduate medicine would be transformed, and so would the quality of patient care, if instead, at least for educational supervisors, the equivalent of the traditional PG Cert were required, and paced appropriately over several years, with a practical teaching component based on the course members current practical responsibilities and debate and discussion of the kinds of topics offered in this book. Such a qualification or equivalent is, after all, required for teaching in most other professions and would enable the development of sound teachers whose educational practice was informed by an understanding of what makes for educationally worthwhile practice.

Supervisors could begin to lay the basis for this by working systematically through many of the topics offered in this book (and others), and by seeking to develop a recognition of the kind of enterprise that education is. Portfolio evidence of their efforts in this respect could be offered as part of the course assessment. The understanding thus developed would surely then lead to a more thoughtful approach to their own teaching, which itself would be further developed if explored carefully and shared with like-minded colleagues. By reading and thinking, they would meet the wisdom enshrined in the traditions and literature of teaching as a profession and learn to aspire to a principled autonomy in which they become their own agents as teachers, because they have developed confidence based on understanding the nature of education and know how to reflect upon, and develop what they offer their learners.

Aspirations for your journey

The details discussed above are now offered in diagrammatic detail in *Figure 2.2 The mountain of educational practice: detail,* which should be read beside *Table 2.1 Towards educational* praxis. This summarises the key points made about each part of the mountain. Readers will note that in order to emphasize the relationship between Figure 2.2 and Table 2.1, coloured text is used in the first column of the Table to match the colours found in the Figure. Both pages should be read from the bottom upwards.

Figure 2.2 The mountain of educational practice: detail

EDUCATION

Engaging in *praxis* as a life-long journey

↑

3. Understanding the nature of *praxis*

Being an educator engaging in the practice of education

↑

2. Understanding the nature of education and self as a person and an educator

Being a teacher engaging in the practice of teaching

↑

I. Thinking like a teacher

EDU-ACTION

iii. Using *ad hoc* random elements of 'theory'

ii. Doing what teachers appear to do

i. Following tips for teachers

TRAINING
Adhering to the elements of Training the Trainers

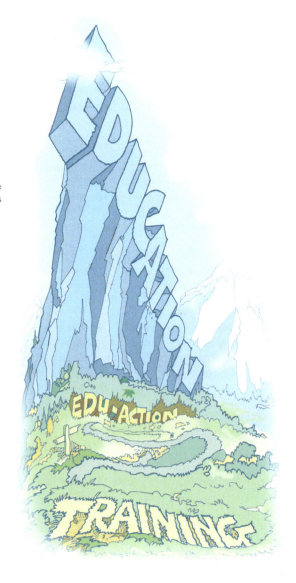

Table 2.1 Towards educational *praxis*

Aspiring to principled autonomy: developing enhanced teaching where teacher is their own educational agent	
Engaging in praxis as a life-long journey. **3. Understanding the nature of *praxis***	Is committed to seeking wisdom. Uses practical reasoning to seek the best for the given learner. Recognizes that education is a moral and intellectual endeavour, where achieving the best for the learner is engaged in for its own sake and not for any other reward. Is endlessly exploring the gamut of educational choices available.
Being an educator engaging in educational practice **2. Understanding the nature of education as a practice and self as a person and a professional**	Can analyze what these learners need (not just want), has an active personal philosophy, sees practice as based on deep educational understanding and professional judgement (how best to act in this situation). Thinks like an educator. Begins to understand self more deeply and develop own character as a teacher. Is own agent.
	Knows about education as well as about teaching. Is aware of own values, has an informed view of what is educationally worthwhile, and recognizes the problematic nature of education. Recognizes that teaching is a moral enterprise with huge responsibilities. Develops, records and keeps under review own personal educational philosophy, and critiques and shares it..
Being a teacher who engages in the practice of teaching **1. Thinking like a teacher**	Makes and implements decisions about how to teach, based on some theoretical understanding about the process of teaching, has growing experience, because well-informed about teaching *as a practice*, and thinks like a teacher. Not very aware that teaching is at core a moral enterprise, and that education is a complex concept.
	Knows some skills and strategies that teachers use and when, where and why to use them. Knows how to get learners to learn, but does not have own personal basis for teaching. Has thought about teaching but not about self as a teacher.
Edu-action: teaching is a loosely-connected set of *ad hoc* actions and teacher is someone else's agent	
iii. Using *ad hoc* random elements of theory	Has attended courses on some 'theory' that is related to educational practice, but has not brought these together into a holistic view of teaching. Does not know the theoretical basis of teaching or how to theorize own practice.
ii. Doing what teachers appear to do	Recognizes some key practical issues about how to get learners to learn, but goes through the motions of these in practice, using own best teacher as a model.
i. Following tips for teachers	Follows some commonsense rules, so general as to be useless and dangerous because they can leave the teacher stranded.
Teaching is not seen as a moral enterprise and teacher is someone else's agent	
Training: adhering to the requirements of Training the Trainers	Goes through a *given* teaching routine automatically and does not engage the minds of learners beyond the basic activity to be learnt.

Where this way of thinking comes from: what Aristotle can teach us

The source of this way of thinking is to be found in the work of Aristotle, and has been usefully explored by Carr, W. (2009). As Wilf Carr shows, the distinction we now make between 'theory' and 'practice' was for Aristotle a three-way distinction between theoretical, technical and practical forms of reasoning. Each of these had an aim (*telos*) which resulted in a different form of reasoning. These are, respectively, to seek truth; to produce a pre-planned artifact; and to do what is wisest in a specific practical situation. This last is a moral commitment to wise action. These aims each arise from different dispositions: *episteme* is based on the disposition to seek knowledge for its own sake; *techné* is based on the disposition to act in a rule-governed, methodical way; and *phronesis* is based on the disposition to act wisely or prudently in a given practical situation (a virtue for its own sake). Each of these in turn engages us in a particular form of action. These are respectively: *theoria* (contemplative action); *poesis* (instrumental actions which require mastery of narrowly defined knowledge and skills, governed by protocols created to provide the maximum result for a pre-determined outcome); and *praxis* ('morally committed action, guided by what is ethically right and proper, and in which, and through which, our values are given practical expression', Carr, W. 2009:60). *Table 2.2 An Aristotelian classification of* Forms of Reasoning illustrates all this.

Table 2.2 An Aristotelian classification of *Forms of Reasoning*
(Adapted from Carr, W. 2009: 60)

Form of reasoning	Theoretical	Technical	Practical
Disposition	**Episteme** The disposition to seek knowledge for its own sake	**Techné** The disposition to act in a rule-governed way to make a pre-planned artifact	**Phronesis** The disposition to act wisely or prudently in a specific situation
Aim (**telos**)	**To seek truth for its own sake...**	**To produce some object or artifact (like a chair or a house or some thing a craftsperson has made to *a pre-conceived design*).**	**To do what is ethically right and proper in a *particular*, practical situation.**
	Seeking to achieve eternal and pure truth	This would produce craft, but not art	The basis of art which includes craft

Form of action	*Theoria:* contemplative action	*Poesis:* Instrumental action that requires mastery of the knowledge, methods and skills that together constitute technical expertise	*Praxis:* morally committed action in which, and through which, our values are given practical expression
Form of knowing	Philosophy or abstract reasoning	Applied knowing or technical reasoning (Greek craftsmen and artisans applied their knowledge — the principles, procedures and operational methods — to achieve their pre-determined outcome)	Knowledge-in-use or practical reasoning (For example: clinical reasoning; professional judgement; going beyond protocols — in relation to a specific case)

If this illustrates the main shape of the journey towards well-informed educational practice, then what are the finer details of all this? The rest of Part One attempts to provide much of the understanding that a medical educator of postgraduate doctors would need to begin to acquire in order to develop their teaching into 'enhanced teaching'.

The following chapter begins this process by offering a number of perspectives on professional practice which, it argues, is an important starting point for the journey.

Further reading

Carr, D. (2005a) Personal and interpersonal relationships in education and teaching: a virtue ethical perspective, *British Journal of Educational Studies,* Vol. **53** (3): 255-271.

* Carr, D. (2006a) Professional and personal values and virtues in education and teaching, *Oxford Review of Education,* Vol. **32** (2): 171-183.

Kemmis, S. and Smith, T. J. (2008) Chapter One: Personal *Praxis.* In S. Kemmis and T.J. Smith (eds) *Enabling Praxis: Challenges for Education.* Rotterdam: Sense Publishers.

Chapter Three

Seeing professional practice anew: exploring the nature of education and medicine

> Whilst writing this chapter, I was unexpectedly involved, as a patient, in two surgical procedures, one of which turned out to be longer and more complex than either I or the surgeon involved expected. I had chosen to see this consultant, whom I had not met before, privately, in order to be able to fit what I needed from her around my professional commitments. Naturally, I paid a fee for what she did, which I regard as fair remuneration for her technical expertise, and as, in one sense, no different from payments I might make at the point of need for any appropriate service I received, whether from a professional or a tradesperson.
>
> But, I also took her a present. This I saw as a response not to her technical expertise but to the *person she is*, which had emerged clearly even in such a short time, through the way she met and responded to me, from the way she conducted herself and inter-related with me during the unexpected demands of the surgery, and in her reaction to my own relief at some good news. Here she went beyond 'duty' and 'obligation' and met me, whole person to whole person.

Introduction
Clarifying some terms: 'practice' and 'professional practice'
Rival conceptions of the nature of professional practice
The nature of practice in medicine and how we might construe it
The nature of practice in education and how we might construe it
Modes of practice in education and medicine
Last words
Further reading

Introduction

In setting out seriously on the demanding journey towards becoming medical educators, the first 'taken-for-granted' ideas that we need to examine more closely and formulate more accurately are about the nature of the professional practices of both medicine and education. This is because how we see the former shapes the kind of doctor we will be trying to cultivate and how we see the latter will become the very bases of all our aspirations, thoughts and actions as a teacher. Thus these matters are an unavoidable starting point for developing a well-founded and well-argued philosophy both for individual medical educators and for PGME itself.

Medicine including surgery, and education, are professional practices. The commonsense view of the nature of medicine is that it is a technical and evidence-based practice, informed by science and performed by knowledgeable and skilful doctors. Montgomery (2006), however, characterizes this as the myth doctors sell to themselves publicly, whilst privately in their actual practice, relying on a far more complex view of medicine! An educator who accepts unthinkingly this common and commonsense view, will expect PGME simply to focus on the acquisition and development of skills and knowledge. Indeed, this is the instrumental thrust of all current curricula for postgraduate medicine. However, a few seconds review of this in the light of what doctors actually do in practice, will show that this seriously underplays what medical practice demands of doctors, and that whilst such curricula properly require such necessary knowledge and skills to be learnt, this alone is by no means sufficient to cover all that teachers need to work on with learning doctors.

Likewise, the practice of teaching is commonly seen as a relatively simple process requiring the teacher to be knowledgeable in content (which is not a problem in PGME), and to be able to exercise a few teaching skills and strategies in order to 'get that content over'. As we shall see, this is an impoverished and outmoded view of what is involved in learning, because, as educators know, 'telling someone' by no means guarantees their understanding. (See, for example, the work of Carr, D.; Carr, W.; Dewey; Freire; Hanson; Oakeshott; Van Manen, M.; and Wells.) There are even more misunderstandings about education than about medicine, because we often slip into unchallenged assumptions that we know what teaching involves and what the practice of education is all about, having been taught by well-prepared and knowledgeable teachers who *appear* to perform smoothly on the simple basis of their knowledge and a few teaching strategies. The assumption therefore, is that anyone can teach as long as they are knowledgeable and possess a few commonsense skills. But again, a few seconds thought will remind us of some who were knowledgeable, but couldn't.

This chapter therefore seeks to foster a structured exploration of the real nature of professional practice in medicine and education. It does so in four sections, starting with some issues about professional practice generally, before focusing down on the specific nature of medical and educational practice. Thus, we begin by exploring ideas about, and clarifying some terms related to, 'practice' and what we mean by 'professional' practice. In the second section we look at the *nature* of professional practice itself, by exploring ideas that lie at the very roots of educating professionals as seen in two contrasting modes of practising as a professional. In the light of these modes of practice, the third section offers some thoughts about the nature of medical practice and how we might construe it, while the fourth looks at the practice of education in these terms.

Clarifying some terms: 'practice' and 'professional practice'

In order to clarify ideas that will be captured by certain terms used in this book, this section considers what we might mean by 'a practice', and then by the word professional in the phrase 'professional practice'. It finally proceeds to look at the traditions of practice in a profession and to explore what is involved in learning in a community of practice.

What is 'a practice'?

The word 'practice', as Golby and Parrott explain, can be used in two major ways in courses of professional preparation (whatever the specific profession involved). It can refer to the *individual activity* or activities of a single practitioner. But, in the term 'professional practice', it is also used to refer to what they have called a 'living tradition' which 'has its own distinctive aims and values' where what people do is intelligible only by reference to (a) their own understandings of what they are doing and (b) the tradition of conduct of which they are a part, (Golby and Parrott 2002: 9). For education, they note, the social project is the promotion of knowledge, just as for the legal profession it is justice and for the medical profession it is health. Using an analogy from everyday life, they helpfully go on to argue that the professional's activities in practice are best understood from within the tradition of professional practice to which they are related. They are at best: temporary; can never be fully solved; are situation specific; are essentially contestable (because value-related); and have a moral dimension. They argue that:

> A practice exists whenever a more or less settled body of activities is carried on to some distinctive end. Activities may be regarded as particular things people do to some overall social purpose. For example, parenthood is a practice (and motherhood and fatherhood too). Within these practices particular activities have their place, a place which may be more or less settled or agreed.
>
> *(Golby and Parrott 2002: 3)*

They cite bedtime routines, methods of discipline, family holidays and excursions, and visits to grandparents as examples of activities which, taken together, give a character to individual parents' practice of parenting. This enables parenting to become something we can talk about, for example, as 'loving' or 'cold', 'permissive' or 'highly disciplined', evidence for this coming from examples of particular activities pursued by the parents in question. Citing the differences in the role of the father in Victorian times and fathers now, they note that 'conventional wisdom about practices changes over time'. Thus, as they show, in engaging in our own practice as a parent, we also contribute to the more general practice of parenting, and such a contribution, they add slightly mischievously but very seriously, is one that makes itself felt most in the subsequent influence it has on our grown-up children and *their* own practice of parenthood. (See Golby and Parrott 2002: 3-4.) This is a solemn reminder of the long-term significance of our educational endeavours.

This is not, however, the same as assuming that when you have listed all the possible activities, knowledge and skill that make up 'a practice', you have summed up what is involved in that practice. It is unwise to extrapolate from this to claim to be able to lay down all that will be needed by everyone on every occasion. That approach to characterizing a job works only where the job requires training as an apprentice, or following a rulebook. But it does not work well for professionals who have to make complex decisions and professional judgements wherever the protocols run out. In professional practice this occurs frequently, because professionals serve individuals each of whom is in some sense unique.

All this demonstrates why 'good practice' cannot consist of simple pre-specifiable skills and activities, as argued for example by Jessup (1991) who was a leading theorist of skills-centred training, and as found in the competencies listed in most modern curricula of most professions. This view misleadingly assumes that breaking down the explicit aspects of a profession's job into every visible component will provide a formula (the sum of those skills) that will produce 'good' professional.

'Being a professional' will always involve more than a simple sum of the parts. It is possible (and perhaps desirable) to require a basic level of practice, that is a just-acceptable standard for entry to a profession, by setting out a list of skills and knowledge required, and using an inspection and control system to enforce just this. But at postgraduate level, in a professional practice, such imposition is anti-educational, amoral and very un-emancipatory, as well as being difficult to police. It is also de-motivating for all those who are well capable of far more than what is on the list! It is a very technical solution to the problem of establishing a basis for cultivating good professionals and remediating poor ones or dispensing with their services.

But the most fundamental flaw in all this is that good practice is *context specific*, can only be described in terms of principle, and is only achieved *in* practice (dialectically and empirically). This also means that good practice cannot be 'mandated' by decree from outside. (No individual's practice can be rendered excellent by trying to 'inspect quality into' it!) As this book is attempting to show, there are better ways to think about all this and sounder and more educational ways of developing good professionals in practice.

What do we mean by 'professional' in the phrase 'professional practice'?

As Golby argues, learning to become a professional is: 'a matter of coming ever more fully into membership of a tradition of practice' and, 'at its maturity it is a matter of taking part in more fully shaping practice for the future'. This involves understanding the inherited traditions of a profession and considering critically and practically their present relevance. (See Golby 1993: 8.)

Professional practice, as Golby points out:

> is not merely habitual skilled behaviour but a stream of highly miscellaneous activities unified as serving a social good. Practice has a history which can be seen as the collective pursuit of human good; as an historic phenomenon, practices have their own language and style. Though there are of necessity routine and unreflecting parts of daily professional life, loss of sight of fundamental values which have evolved historically in the activities of practice is at once a loss of professionalism.
>
> *(Golby 1993: 5)*

For the current purpose, we need to note that in this book the term professional is used to define practice as something engaged in by a *member* of a profession. (See Fish and Coles (2005), chapter five, for full details of what this involves). It is also something one is and one lives, rather than a mere label to indicate the group one belongs to.

It follows that in postgraduate medicine, teachers should provide learners with a range of possible ways of construing the kind of professional they are and wish to become and the kind of professional practice they wish to engage in. For resources to aid discussions about professionalism with learning doctors see Fish and de Cossart (2007) chapter five; and Cruess, Creuss and Steinert (2008). *Frame 3.1 Some comments about professionalism*, offers three quotations that might be useful as starting points for teachers and learners to consider. It should be noted that all three raise important issues about how doctors should, *as professionals*, conduct themselves.

Frame 3.1 Some comments about professionalism

'We take professionals to be persons who seek a broad understanding of their practice, paying attention not only to their developing competence, but also to the fundamental purposes and values that underpin their work'.

Prof Michael Golby, Exeter University

'Professionalism is an aspect of practice that is assessed in all doctors from the Foundation Years to the end of specialty training. It is significant in shaping the relationships with all other healthcare colleagues. It is recognised by the sick as central to the quality of their care, and is a crucial element in patients' attitudes to their doctors....
It is therefore important that doctors in training be enabled to explore, defend and critique the key principles and values to which they aspire and which they intend to use to shape their working lives.

Profs Della Fish and Linda de Cossart, Chester University

'A good professional has to be someone who possesses, in addition to specified theoretical or technical expertise, a range of distinctly moral attitudes, values and motives designed to elevate the interests and needs of clients, patients or pupils above self-interest.'

David Carr, Emeritus Professor, Edinburgh University

It will readily be seen that in all these comments, the hallmarks of a professional go well beyond mere expertise in knowledge and skill. Medical educators will need to have formulated their ideas about this, because these will become the bases of their educational aims as teachers, and these aims will shape everything that they offer in the name of education.

It is also important to recognize that in joining a practice which like all practices will have developed over time, a learning doctor will need help from a teacher or teachers in making sense of their working context. The following two sub-sections seek to lay the underpinning foundations of understanding in respect of this.

The traditions of practice in a profession

When we work as a professional we are always acting within — or in response to — the traditions of our practice. This refers to the ways of doing things and of thinking about things that 'are the norm' because they have come to characterize our profession. They have developed over time until the present. (Such development is of course often not linear and not always for the best!) Many of these 'traditional ways of doing things' are the tacit but accepted norms of life in that social group, such that they do not need to be referred to, because they are the 'done thing' that everyone knows about. These traditions are what give complexity and richness to the everyday life of professionals. They shape and give meaning to the situated lived experiences of people like doctors, teachers, and lawyers, all of whom work as professionals with vulnerable patients, learners and clients, and make decisions with and about them. Such work lies in the realm of moral practice.

Examples of the kinds of aspects of practice that capture the range of what is involved in the traditions of that practice include those in *Table 3.1 Some constituents of the traditions of practice.*

Table 3.1   Some constituents of the traditions of practice

Activities	Agreements	Arrangements
Expectations	Frameworks	Habits
Informing theories	Inventions	Logic
Practice ontology	Priorities	Relationships
Routines	Rules	Systems
Tacit understandings	Values	What is and what isn't negotiable

The significance of all this for the teacher of professionals, of course, is to what extent they are responsible for inculcating the norms of the profession into their learners, and to what extent they should encourage criticality, flexibility and more creative thinking. As Benjamin's famous myth 'The Sabre-tooth Curriculum' shows us, (Benjamin 1931) it also raises several interesting dilemmas.

▷ Is one's responsibility as a teacher to en-culture learners into an unthinking acceptance of the *present* traditions of practice in their profession?

▷ To what extent and in what ways, as a teacher, should our personal views about practice in our profession colour and shape what and how we teach?

▷ How, as teachers, should we construe, and how should we encourage learning professionals to construe, the significance of the community of practice within which the professional is working?

These are all moral matters for the teacher that need careful and frequent consideration and review. As we shall see further below, how we respond to them will depend on how, as teachers, we see the nature of education.

How new members of a profession learn these 'norms' is also an interesting issue. Many of them are learnt through and as part of being a member of a community that inevitably learns together in practice. However, this does not absolve the teacher from taking a view about such learning and from acting as guide to the learner in not taking for granted as appropriate all the behaviour that is seen and heard in the practice setting, but rather considering it critically and engaging in it thoughtfully. Thus, doctors learn to practise not merely by being told what to do and how to do it by their teachers. They learn within and from their communities of practice, and their teachers need to understand this too.

Learning in a community of practice

As Wenger (1998) points out, our identity as practitioners is shaped by: the way we talk about our changing abilities; how we see our shared historical and social frameworks; how we participate in the social configurations that confirm our competence; and how we understand the changes that result from our learning.

He then argues that learning in practice includes the following processes for the communities involved:

> *evolving forms of mutual engagement;* (discovering how to engage with co-workers, and what helps and what hinders developing mutual relationships; defining identities; establishing who is who, who is good at what, who knows what, who is easy or hard to get along with)
>
> *understanding and tuning their enterprise;* (aligning their engagement with it, learning to become and hold each other accountable to it, struggling to define what the enterprise is all about)
>
> *developing their repertoire, styles and discourses;* (renegotiating the meaning and importance of various elements, recalling events, inventing new terms, creating and breaking routines).
>
> *(Summarised from Wenger 1998: 5)*

Wenger sees these three dimensions of learning as interdependent and interlocked into a tight system. Medical educators need to take some account of this and open up their learners to such wider awareness.

It would, of course, be easy to dismiss the need for thinking about this range of issues, as matters resting on mere 'common sense' — something to be taken for granted and not worth dwelling on, given that there are patients needing treatment. However, all so-called common sense is in fact grounded in a set of unrecognized, and thus unexplored views, which themselves are *theories* about what is important and about how things are or should be done. (See, for example, Smith, 1992.) It is arguable therefore that the medical educator's responsibility is to develop doctors and surgeons as full and fully-aware members of their profession. In order to do so, they will need to bring such issues — and those that now follow — to the attention of their learners. Indeed, as postgraduate doctors, it is their basic educational entitlement to be supported by their teachers in exploring all these issues (many of which were natural topics for discussion when 'trainees' met regularly, and learnt within, their firm).

Rival conceptions of the nature of professional practice

This section draws on the work of David Carr (Carr, 2003; 2004) in examining two contrasting ways of thinking about and engaging in professional practice (the technical and the moral mode), and what they each mean for the everyday practice of doctors and the educational responsibilities of their teachers.

The technical mode of practice is engaged in by those professionals who see their job as a matter of dealing with technical problems by providing technical solutions through expertise that depends more or less exclusively on specialist knowledge and relevant skills. In short, they see those they provide for, not so much as *people*, but as technical problems. This assumes that the world in which they work is scientific, objective, and largely mechanistic and well ordered, such that the application of knowledge and skill is a fairly straightforward matter. The aim of a medical educator who thought like this would be to seek to produce a doctor who was a skilled and knowledgeable performer who could solve technical problems effectively and efficiently.

By contrast to this, the moral mode of practice sees the professional as someone who brings their knowledge and skill to the whole person they serve, by relating to them, person to person, with all the human and moral responsibilities that this brings. They also see the world as complex, unpredictable and not yielding so simply to the application of theoretical knowledge and pre-learnt skills. Such a doctor would need from their teachers, in addition to a focus on knowledge and skills, support and nurturing in the development of their character, personal qualities, professional judgement, humane understanding and the flexibility and courage to persist in the face of difficulties.

As we shall see, these contrasting ways of conceptualizing professionals' practice bring with them different concepts, identified through contrasting language, that shape professionals' whole way of seeing the world of their work.

David Carr points out very clearly that there is 'a significant difference between technical and moral modes of practical engagement with the world [but that] almost any human activity is likely to have both moral and technical dimensions or implications'. However, he adds:

> there are nevertheless crucial differences between senses of 'good' as used to qualify character and skilled performance, and between the ways in which goodness of personhood and goodness of technique are measured and fostered.
>
> *(Carr, D. 2004: 106)*

Thus, for example, in the technical mode of practice, 'good practice' is about 'delivering' a performance using pre-set skills, strategies and book-knowledge or formal theory. Here, the question about what makes a good teacher (or doctor), is usually responded to by listing as evidence a vast number of competencies or skills that are observable and countable, and pointing to a syllabus which lists all the knowledge they should know. This is then expected to cash out into success for the learner, evidenced through 'assessment tools' which are seen as separate from teaching and learning, and which measure the observable and treat that which cannot be observed as trivial. The problem here is that although these things are countable, they cannot be *counted on* to tell us everything about 'quality'. Their sum does not automatically amount to the whole 'good' that we seek for either teacher or learner!

Further, the practitioner who works in the technical mode of practice is merely the agent of — and has yielded sovereignty in a number of areas to — others outside their practice (administrators, bureaucrats, regulators, even politicians). For example a teacher holding this view naturally abdicates to others the responsibility for:

▷ *what should be taught* (the curriculum on paper is seen as 'to be obeyed' not as a guide which needs endless development)

▷ *what makes 'good practice'* (the list of skills / competencies and knowledge is accepted as decreed by someone outside the practice context)

▷ *what is the 'right thing to do'* (the only moral compass we need is seen as obedience to 'the rules' which are treated as absolute and sufficient law).

This way of seeing it converts practice into a kind of applied science or theory-based approach that casts practitioners into the role of technician, and construes professional effectiveness largely as performances of measurable skills. This view is currently highly prevalent, and as Carr, D. (2004) says, it is a view that has been considerably overplayed in the last two decades. It would also seem to be a flawed way of seeing professional practice, since many attributes that are characterized as skills are not skills at all, and would probably be better understood and developed when seen as capacities. An example would be professional judgement.

By contrast to all this, in the moral mode of practice, the good practitioner is constituted of more than knowledge and skills (epistemology). Here, *the person the practitioner is* radically affects what they do and can achieve (with say learners or patients). This emphasizes the ontological dimensions of practice, such that a good practitioner is seen as one who:

▷ possesses moral awareness about their practice responsibilities

▷ establishes a human and humane mode of engagement with clients

▷ is an agent of their own practice because they take responsibility for all aspects of it, and make wise choices about what to do, which may be guided, but are not constrained, by national requirements (by the curriculum if they are teachers — or by protocols if they are doctors).

In the moral mode of practice, the practitioner knows and can make clear their own values, recognizing them as driving their thinking, and has the discretion (exercised with principled autonomy) to make wise judgements for and about the learner / patient in the light of their specific context and their particular needs. In all this, the kind of human being they are, as both a person and a professional practitioner, matters, because they seek to meet the whole learner or patient with the whole of themselves in order to work in their service. Such practitioners develop an understanding of *how to 'be'* with that learner / patient, which is about developing character and personality attuned perceptively and affectively to the moral aspects of the practice experience, and is not about *appearing* to behave like a good practitioner — a demeanour that, ironically, is quickly recognized by both learners and patients!

In this mode of practice, for example, a teacher: is finely tuned to the learner; can support and challenge them; can probe and develop their thinking and moral perspectives; and will attend both to the learner's developing *conduct* (action driven by acknowledged principles and articulated values) and to their character or *personhood*, rather than simply their *behaviour* (action driven by an outside agent rather than by the understanding and conviction of the learner).

The education of a learning doctor under this view, would focus as key concerns, not simply on routine medical skills and knowledge, but crucially also on:

▷ that doctor's understanding and knowledge of themselves as a doctor

▷ their sensitivity to the particularities and humanity of each patient

▷ their ability to establish a therapeutic relationship with each patient

▷ their awareness that their interpretation of the context(s) in which they meet the patient will profoundly shape their clinical decisions in this case

▷ their capacity for sound and rigorous clinical thinking

▷ their capacity for making wise professional judgements that are not compromised by self-interest

▷ their ability to see beyond the immediate in weighing up the clinical choices available in each case.

Such an agenda might thus offer the learner new ways of thinking and of being, that challenge the status quo of what we might call 'old-style medical education' where teaching is characterized as telling the learner 'the knowledge', where assessment is about counting the learner's skills, and where clinical practice conforms uncritically to protocols. There, 'the given' in medical practice (the current reality of clinical work and its context) is unquestioningly accepted and obeyed. An example would be simply accepting the need to prioritize the demands of clinical work to the point where there was very little if any time for any serious and in-depth education.

These principles of two very different ways of construing practice go back to Aristotle and have been well-recognized by many educationists since — particularly those in the last twenty years who wish to characterize quality teaching and learning in ways other than through competencies, but whose voice has until now been mainly excluded from public debate. (See, for example: Carr, D. 2004; Carr, W. 1995; Cruess, Cruess and Steinert 2008; Dunne 1995; 2005; and Fish and Brigley 2010). If medical education is to move forward it needs to recognize these ideas and work to ensure their implementation.

Indeed, one key insight associated with the moral mode of practice (whether it be educational or medical), is that in order to aspire to change the world for the better in some way (to offer understanding, enlightenment and emancipation; or cure, treatment or palliation) *we have first to change ourselves in respect of becoming agents of our own moral stance instead of being obedient to convention.*

Thus, a moral response, as illustrated by Carr, D. is to:

> get to the bottom of things, and getting to the moral bottom of things is above all a matter of making *myself* more honest, courageous, self-controlled, just, caring, and so on.
>
> [This] is a matter of ... personal change or development on the part of agents, not just of behaviour modification or increase in intellectual knowledge: and such change of heart can be a function of nothing less than coming to see the value of virtue for its own sake...
>
> *(Carr, D. 2004: 107)*

he adds later that:

> such development of self and others involves the reflective refining or enhancement of conduct in complex contexts of human association...
>
> *(Ibid: 110-11)*

So, as postgraduate medical educators, then, how do we wish to construe the practices of medicine and of education? The next section offers some thoughts on the nature of *medicine* as a practice and how we might construe it within the moral mode of practice, while the final section looks at the practice of *education*.

The nature of practice in medicine and how we might construe it

How might we characterize current medical practice? The following points have in my experience resonated with many doctors who work 'on the ground' within the NHS. They have been adapted from Fish and Coles (2005).

▷ The reality of the lived clinical experience for doctors is more multi-faceted than simply being about getting the patient better and requires more than textbook knowledge, and the ability to carry out laid down procedures and technical skills.

▷ Medicine involves, lying beneath the overall categories of differential diagnosis / treatment plans / care pathways, the real detail — the need for important medical abilities and capacities and for personal-professional characteristics and qualities that go well beyond having and applying traditional knowledge and skills.

▷ Medical practice requires many immediate and highly informed judgements to be made by the doctor with and on behalf of vulnerable and sometimes confused patients, often on the spot and in collaboration with fellow professionals. But judgement is not 'a skill'. It cannot be taught by a lecture-presentation to learners. It can only be nurtured over time through rigorous and deep reflection on experiences in which judgement has been central.

▷ In addition to traditional knowledge and skills, medical practice demands of doctors a wise mixture of intuition, professional on-the-spot judgement, hunch, and risk-taking. Such wisdom cannot be learnt from a textbook or taught directly. It can only be cultivated over a period of time through professional conversations in which specific cases are reflected upon deeply and from which only working principles can be drawn. This is because principles will travel and will guide practice in other similar circumstances, but learnt skills and knowledge cannot be simply applied in every case. Rather they have to be adapted to each new context — as guided by the sound principles gained through reflection on experience.

▷ All medical practice is informed by esoteric and complex procedural and propositional knowledge, but this needs to be shaped by recognition of the moral dimensions of working with and for patients and colleagues, (as controlled through the traditional professional parameters for shaping proper conduct, and influenced by the need for accountability).

▷ Complex medical practice is difficult to learn except through rigorous reflection on specific experience, and even then, although one can illuminate the knowledge embedded in a piece of professional practice, one often cannot fully express in plain words all that has been demanded of the doctor. Metaphors sometimes come to the rescue here, but talking at this deep level can only occur within a nurturing and trusting relationship between teacher and learner.

▷ In many senses such medical practice involves creativity, and is based upon practical wisdom (which comes from more than mere accrued and repeated experience but which evolves through experience that has been rigorously explored by means of reflection until the deeper understanding of that practice has been achieved).

▷ It is about communicating with and working with immediate colleagues, and the multi-professional team, and knowing and being able to assess one's own strengths and weaknesses.

▷ Ironically, the propositional (factual) health-care knowledge called upon in any doctor's individual interaction with patients is often a small proportion of medical knowledge as a whole. It is necessary to know as much of it as possible, and to know when to use it, but such knowledge is actually one of many resources, all of which need a place in the curriculum for practice.

▷ Doctors are individual members of a range of professional communities, in each of which they have responsibilities to their fellows. This makes medical practice (and learning it) a social and collaborative enterprise. Such professional communities include, for example, the community of the work-place; of one's specialist knowledge; of one's professional body; and of professions generally.

▷ Such qualities, characteristics and understandings cannot (except in trivial matters) be satisfactorily categorized in boxes or assessed via tick lists and one-page forms.

In de Cossart and Fish (2005) we summed this up by saying:

> [Professionals] endlessly create, negotiate and develop meanings; have to be appropriately flexible about some things and temporarily inflexible about others; engage all the time with multiple activities, factors, and perspectives; ceaselessly formulate problems and solutions; and learn to live with, the insoluble, the ephemeral, the tentative and the incomplete.
>
> *(de Cossart and Fish 2005: 100)*

Young doctors working in the 21st century need this understanding developed in them, together with wise judgement, in order to make themselves and their patients safe — especially in a world in which patients now have the same access to medical knowledge that doctors do (via the internet) but who may well not fully understand how best to tailor it to their own case.

But there is more to be said. The thesis informing this book (as it also informed Fish 2010) is that both *practising interpretively* and its basis, *practical reasoning*, already exist in medicine but with little explicit recognition, and that they urgently need to be nurtured by means of wise medical education. Practical reasoning or *phronesis* and *praxis* or morally committed action (as we saw in chapter two, pp. 40-41 above), are what the professional engages in so as to make wise judgements in situations of uncertainty. It is the need for such decisions, hour by hour in practice, which makes medicine not a technical practice but an interpretive one. Medical educators who understand this are in the best position to develop wise doctors.

Montgomery highlights the inaccurate avowal of doctors that they practise according to evidence-based medicine. She attributes this to 'a field defect in their vision of themselves and their practice', which she says causes them:'publicly to "misdescribe" their practice as rule-governed and evidence-based', when in fact the way they work shows medicine to be substantially interpretive. (See Montgomery 2006: 5.) As I argued several years later:

> An unfortunate result of this is that as long as the real nature of that practice (their practical reasoning) remains largely tacit, it cannot be understood, explored and developed, thus depriving beginners of gaining an explicit introduction to it and mature professionals of developing it further.

I also suggested that the result of medicine being an interpretive practice is that:

This requires professionals (through education) to become explicitly aware of their own values and how these drive their interpretations of practice, even as they engage in it. This in turn enables them to develop further their ability to interpret wisely the complexities of a particular patient's healthcare needs. It also requires them, in the light of this, to formulate and then exercise professional judgment, thus acting with discretion on the patient's behalf, and so recognising and fulfilling their moral responsibilities to the patient.

I added:

The role of education here is to empower professionals to become more explicit about their tacit practical rationality and more conscious of their values and capacities, so that they can refine and develop them, and can be articulate about their significance in best patient care. In short, through education they become more fully the operators of their own practice and its development, rather than relying solely on the endless updating of knowledge and skills!

(Fish 2010: 193 - 94)

What does this assume or require, then about the nature of the practice of education?

The nature of practice in education and how we might construe it

Perhaps the most important inference from all this is that educational practice, construed as being a moral practice, should be about the emancipating development of self and others, not about the locking of learners into a narrow and narrowing world of the avaricious acquisition of endless skills, protocols and theoretical knowledge!

Education is essentially a values-based concept. This means that it is, to some degree, problematic and not able to be given a once-for-all definition, simply because people use the terms 'education' and 'educated' in approval of an enterprise or person, and their approval depends on what they value most. Thus we might ask the following. Is the term 'educated' to be reserved only for those with Latin and Greek or does being well-mannered matter more? Are we schooled in educational institutions but educated by life? The problem here is that different people value different aspects of life and therefore of education, so that medical educators work amidst a conflicting set of educational values. Thinking about all this prompts educators to have a view on what educational practice means for them, to seek to nurture learners to understand these complexities, and to choose wisely what kind of a professional they might aspire to become. To be able to articulate this for a range of important audiences and purposes is a vital part of being an educator.

Further, these issues should not be ducked in the name of everything educational being merely 'contestable and therefore never able to be resolved into any kind of consensus'. It is the view of this book that while there are deeply contrasting views about education (because, as we shall see, it is values-based), this does not preclude coming to some general agreements, about a number of important and fundamental matters, in which a range of views can be encompassed and incorporated, to the benefit of all (see Carr, D. 2010).

The importance of values — educational, and indeed, professional

Values are those abiding and long-cherished views we all have — but do not necessarily share — about what counts as enduringly worthwhile and important. These views and values shape our practice, whether we know it or not. They are usually tacit, often lying deep beneath the surface of our practice.

Values are by definition matters of contention, because often they are not shared by other members of our working environment. (It is true that any healthcare professional will share many values with immediate colleagues, but this may not be true across professions, let alone in relation to other staff and to patients.) Indeed, everyone who works in a professional practice lives at the centre of a web of complex, but subtle and largely invisible pressures that arise from the differing values endemic to professional practice and its management, (see de Cossart and Fish 2005: 20).

Values are rarely directly discussed, (so that colleagues do not recognize their differences as values-based), and so the pressures that arise from them are not traced to source and thus become puzzling as well as frustrating. Indeed, contention about values results from seriously different ways of seeing the world, and leads to very different ways of conducting ourselves.

Whether we are aware of it or not, educational values lie at the centre of how we conduct ourselves as teachers, and clinical values are central and fundamental to the professional practice and expertise of doctors. It is thus the unavoidable responsibility of the teacher of postgraduate doctors to have made explicit both sets of values as enshrined in their own practice, and also to recognize that they may espouse some values that they do not manage to attain. That is, as teachers we should begin any attempt to understand and develop any professional practice, both by exploring our own educational values and by recognizing the clinical values we seek to promote. Only then will we be equipped to enable learners to explore their own professional values.

Such an exploration is bound to begin by looking at the visible elements of what a practitioner does, and then attempting to gain access to and understand what drives these. Practitioners rarely talk or write directly about their values, yet, what they do, know and think, speak volumes in respect of what they believe is important. Indeed, ironically, that which practitioners take for granted, and overlook (because it is so much a natural part of their practice), is often very visible to patients, learners and other colleagues who observe them. (See Fish and Coles 2005, chapters three and four.)

Making our educational values explicit as a basis for educational practice

Our *professional* values in general are how we each consistently see the world in which we engage in *professional* practice, and what we prioritize in our professional life. Our professional values are what drive our professional actions, attitudes, thoughts and beliefs. And one's conduct reveals these values to all those one works with (colleagues and patients). Such values existed well before one became conscious of them, and whether one is aware of them or not, they have a profound effect on how others see one. They might also be seen in our views about the ways others engage in practice.

Our educational values shape how we each conduct ourselves as a teacher in the clinical setting. And it should be noted that clinicians working with learners in the clinical setting are *always* teaching their own values (indirectly by modelling, if not explicitly through discussion). Our educational values spring from our own educational experiences which will have shaped how we see the role of the teacher, how we think about teaching as a practice, how we conceive of what learners are like and what they need, and how we envisage assessment as a practice. All this will affect how we each teach and learn and what our learners gain from their time with us.

Sometimes our *actions* as teachers reveal educational values that are different from those we would say we hold. (We might claim to value the learner's views, but how we behave towards them might tell them that we do not!) Here there is a gap between our espoused values (values we claim to hold) and our values-in-use (values that emerge from our practice). Whilst our espoused educational values and our educational values-in-use are in harmony, there is no conflict. But this is rare, and something to strive for rather than something we can easily attain. When we recognize such a values gap, it is always worth exploring further both our practice and our values.

Education as a moral practice

When education is seen as a technical practice, it focuses on the teacher learning a range of skills and strategies for given situations and using them efficiently. When seen as a *moral activity*, it is held to be undertaken in pursuit of *educationally worthwhile ends*, which aim to realize morally worthwhile virtues. Examples of this are as follows.

- ▶ The role of the educator is to facilitate the process of growth in the learner (to enhance individual freedom, develop autonomy and contribute to democracy). See, for example, the work of Dewey.

- ▶ Education liberates individuals and facilitates their transition from passive to active learners. See the work of Carr, W; Oakeshott; Palmer.

- ▶ Education is emancipatory, cannot be morally neutral, and is always directive (but the ends and means used can be liberating). It is a social process and above all it is the practice of freedom in which learners discover themselves and achieve their humanity. See the work of Freire.

As we shall see in chapter four, these worthwhile ends, aims or goals of education include the development of the whole person and particularly the *cultivation of the mind*, which means developing understanding which in turn will lead to the development of practice.

Modes of practice in education and medicine

It is important to explore and clarify the relationships between the technical and the moral modes of practice, and these are expressed below in *Figure 3.1 Understanding modes of practice in medical education: a continuum*.

Here the three cubes depicted represent three ways of construing a teacher's practice, and demonstrate the relationship between these as along a continuum. The left hand cube represents a 'narrow training' view of the technical mode of practice. Here, the focus is strictly and exclusively upon training the trainee in the technical skills and the specifics of the specialist knowledge associated with professional practice. This is the most extreme version of the technical mode of practice and is found in the work of the technical trainer who is concerned only with inculcating change in the trainee's behaviour, so that they adopt, follow and ultimately even teach *protocols* as *the* basis for coping with complex practical problems. This is more appropriate for craft apprentices than for doctors and when used in medicine will result in highly restricted professionals unable to exercise the kind of professional judgement needed by patients.

The middle cube represents the views of the medical teacher working more broadly in the technical mode of practice. But visible behaviour rather than conduct shaped by the learner's values, is still the priority. Here the teacher may be trying to re-shape the learner's behaviour in terms of broader skills that need to become automatic and to inculcate extensive specialist knowledge in the learner. This seems less narrow but still produces technicians who are, arguably, restricted professionals.

The view of professional education represented in the right hand cube is that professional judgement is the central core of professional practice and that developing this in learning doctors requires the teacher to work in the moral mode of practice where the development of the learner's conduct, character and understanding are of priority. Here the teacher aims at developing a holistic doctor who meets patients as one human being to another and can utilize their knowledge, skills, and judgement creatively in their service. Such a doctor is seen as an extended professional.

Perhaps the most important aspect of *Figure 3.1*, is that it indicates the possibility of the teacher moving along this continuum from left to right, and also shows that the right hand cube does not eschew the technical aspects of practice.

Figure 3.1 Understanding modes of practice in medical education: a continuum
(After the work of Carr, D. 2003)

(All modes may be needed but the educated teacher chooses them in an informed way)

Working in the technical mode of practice → **Working in the moral mode of practice**

	Highly restricted professional	Restricted professional	Extended professional
Kind of professional	Working in the technical mode of practice	Working in the technical mode of practice	Working in the moral mode of practice
Kind of practitioner the teacher is	Technical trainer working in the technical mode of practice	Medical teacher working in the technical mode of practice	Medical teacher working in the moral mode of practice
Construes practice as	concerned with **CHANGING behaviour** in which teacher is the agent for inculcating in the doctor procedures pre-determined by a higher authority and where the doctor can only practise by the book	concerned with **SHAPING behaviour** in which teacher is the agent for ensuring that the required procedures and knowledge and where the doctor is only focused on what that teacher requires	concerned with **DEVELOPING conduct** where teacher ensures that the doctor UNDERSTANDS the required procedures and knowledge and how to use them intelligently and nurtures the doctor as a person with their own repertoire of decision-making and who serves the patient
	The narrow face of technical practice	The technical face of professional practice	The moral face of professional practice
Kind of practitioner the learner is	Technical trainee, a follower of protocols	Technician Doctor focused on medical skills and knowledge (the visible aspects of practice)	Holistic Doctor focused on skills and knowledge, nurtured as a person and developing the invisible aspects of practice including professional judgement
Good teaching seen as	A SIMPLE PROCESS, involving *training* in skills that have been well learnt (uncritically) through repetition, have been observed as well performed by an assessor, so that the required change in learners' behaviour will occur on all occasions.	A SIMPLE MATTER OF TELLING clearly, through presentation of teacher's knowledge or skills, (assumed to be easily absorbed by the learner) and thoroughly checked via a rigorously applied 'required' test of a learner's behaviour / knowledge, that most learners pass.	A COMPLEX PROFESSIONAL PRACTICE in which the learner's knowledge, skills, character, capacities, professionalism, decision-making and professional judgement are nurtured by a wide range of means, employed to educationally worthwhile ends.

60

Last words

These ideas are only a starting point and many of them will be explored further in a range of different ways throughout the rest of Part One, whilst Part Two will consider the practical implications of all this, and will offer examples and suggestions for how all this can be translated into practice.

Further reading

* Carr, D. (2004) Rival conceptions of Practice in Education and Teaching, in J. Dunne, and P. Hogan (eds) *Education and Practice: Upholding the Integrity of Learning*. Oxford: Blackwell Publishing: 102-115.

Fish, D. (2010) Learning to Practise Interpretively: exploring and developing practical rationality, in J. Higgs, D. Fish, I. Goulter, S. Loftus, J-A. Reid and F. Trede (eds) *Education for Future Practice*. Rotterdam: Sense Publications: 191-202.

* Montgomery, K. (2006) *How Doctors Think: clinical judgement and the practice of medicine*. Oxford: Oxford University Press.

Chapter Four

Seeing the teacher's responsibilities anew: a view from the moral mode of practice

> The relationship I have with my learner must be honest, non-judgemental and committed. They must trust that I will be patient, flexible and open-minded to engage with them on an equal level so that they feel more empowered to take part more fully in shaping practice for the future.... Medicine is not an easy path and any learner has the right to be nurtured until they are able to go it alone... most importantly, I wish to instill the moral aspect of practice back into the curriculum....
>
> Extract from the personal philosophy, written at the completion of the PG Cert, by one of the consultants whose first observations were referred to in chapter one above.

Introduction
Training and education: key differences in teachers' responsibilities
Teaching as a moral activity: what it means to work in the moral mode of practice
So, in the light of this, what is 'good' teaching?
Further reading

Introduction

The way we see professional practice as teachers and doctors has profound consequences for our daily lives and careers. As the previous chapter shows, professionals who see themselves as technicians, view their practice as relatively simple in nature, requiring from their teachers (who are content to adopt the role of trainer) attention only to their learners' knowledge and skills. In this process, the trainer inculcates in the trainee the necessary changes of behaviour to 'make' them more effective and efficient. Such teachers, or rather trainers, would probably rely for support in this on a list of tips for teachers, as available in many texts on medical education. They would see 'good teachers' as those whose practice was characterized by *their* knowledge and presentational expertise, made visible as a performance, in which they were demonstrably technically effective in changing — in pre-designed ways — the *behaviour* and even the knowledge (but not the understanding) of their learners. Here, the teacher's success is rated against a notional checklist of visible skills, and how much they have changed their learners' behaviour. There is very little intellectual activity in all this and no moral dimension is required. Here, learners become the objects of teaching, and teachers are often mere 'edu-tainers'.

As already demonstrated, however, once examined carefully, professional practice generally and the practices of medicine and education particularly, prove inescapably to be moral practices. This makes very different and more complex demands upon the teacher, calling for an enhanced version of teaching as an educational practice. In this mode, medical teachers recognize the responsibility to attend to the learning doctor's *knowing, doing, thinking, being and becoming*, and they can only do so as a result of having themselves been nurtured and developed *as teachers* in all these dimensions. Here, the good teacher, as Hansen says so clearly, is seen as: 'enriching, not impoverishing, students' understandings of self, others, and the world.... expanding, not contracting, students' knowledge, insight, and interests.... deepening, not rendering more shallow, students' ways of thinking and feeling.' Such a teacher deserves the accolade educator (Hansen 2001: ix).

There are, therefore, key differences in responsibility between trainers and educators. In its first section, this chapter will explore these more fully. This will be followed, in section two, by a focus on teaching as a moral practice, which will try to tease out the responsibilities of a medical teacher working in the moral and complex mode of educational practice in order to educate postgraduate doctors about the finer aspects of being a doctor, as well as to enable them to acquire the knowledge and skills they need. Section three will then offer an overview of what, within this mode, constitutes 'a good teacher'. Equipped with these ideas, we look in the final section at some principles of how teachers working in the moral mode of practice think, and what they consider particularly, as they prepare to interact with their learners, and also how they construe the evaluation processes that will provide them with appropriate data with which to reflect seriously on their own practice in order to develop and improve it.

Training and education: key differences in teachers' responsibilities

The terms 'education' and 'training' often lie unexplored beneath the term 'teaching'. Indeed ironically, the term 'training' is often casually employed in postgraduate medicine, by supervisors who actually describe their work as training when in fact they are engaging in education! When this happens, it shows that the teacher has not fully grasped what they are actually about. It can also offer the learner mixed messages. Clarity on the teacher's part about the vastly contrasting differences between the values, concepts and activities of training, and of education, is an essential basis for optimizing the time spent with learners. This is because it dramatically affects how the teacher sees their responsibilities to the learner — and beyond the learner to their profession — and shapes how the learner both regards and relates to the teacher.

Teachers as trainers

Teachers as trainers — even of postgraduate professionals — see themselves working with 'workers', who need to become more efficient and effective in order to fulfil better their current role or take on greater responsibility in their job. Such trainers see themselves as having a responsibility to act unquestioningly as the agent of various higher authorities, to equip workers with visibly greater knowledge and more advanced skills, it is assumed, they will automatically apply directly to and within their daily work. The problem here is that very little of what is learnt during such training can be applied directly by professionals who work in contexts that are never the same twice, (as compared with factory-workers who produce standard widgets all day). The trainers' preparation for fulfilling this function will, of course, have involved being trained!

Training involves ensuring that the same reaction is always given to a similar event —without the need to pause for thought. Soldiers train in order unthinkingly to obey orders instantly in emergency events. Children (and other learners) are trained in certain behavioural matters in order to establish unconscious rituals and habits that will keep them safe and help them learn. Surgeons train in 'basic surgical skills' in order to familiarize them with key sensory knowledge and establish certain surgical routines that will help to ensure patients' safety and well-being.

Training is often provided in a one-off session, and frequently is aimed at rehearsing learners in protocols. The notion of development over time is not central to the trainer's responsibilities. Training seeks to dispense with thought and to engage trainees in unquestioning and automatic response to certain situations. These activities also assume a clear hierarchy between trainer and trainee, such that engaging the trainee in discussion does not feature large within a trainer's list of key responsibilities. Neither is the trainer required to engage the learner in debating wider educational issues. Thus trainees learn 'how' to do something but not 'why', 'when', 'when not' and 'where' and 'where not' to do it. Nor are trainers expected to encourage the learner to bring wider critical perspectives to bear either on the planned ends and means that drive the training session, or on its actual outcome.

It may be true that a very small amount of professional practice involves trained rituals but even these can be dangerous to a client/patient if they are used without questioning how appropriate their use is in the given context. In fact, most of the activities a member of a profession carries out need to be underpinned by education, not training. This will inevitably raise issues about moral and ethical matters.

The terms ethical and moral

The term 'ethical', here, is taken to mean 'that which is accepted as the norms of any group or society'. In any group or profession, ethical norms help people to act decently in given situations (to act or do 'good' or 'the right' as opposed to perpetrating 'the bad' or 'the wrong'). The means of establishing these is through well-argued philosophical debate and reference to the classical, the Christian and other spirituals virtues. This is quite different from talking about what is 'correct and incorrect' or 'valid and invalid', which relate to arbitrarily agreed standards that use empirical means to evidence them through measurement. The norms in any group or society or profession include formal and codified standards and also informally agreed ones that set out the boundaries of how members of the group should conduct themselves. It should be remembered of course that even within one profession, the practitioner is actually a member of a number of groups, each of which will have its own norms. Also, the norms are not 'handed down from above', but arise and develop as the group or profession evolves. They are the traditions of practice.

The term moral, relates to 'morality', which is taken to mean an individual's relationship with the ethics of the group to which they belong. Particularly it is about the degree to which an individual conforms to (agrees with and acts according to) the moral law or ethics of their group. Sometimes in following a set of ethics of one subgroup to which we belong, we transgress those of another. Sometimes we have to have the courage to stand out against an aspect of current ethics that do not conform to what we personally believe is good. This is particularly true for doctors, for example, when they see the need to step outside the norms of a protocol or a set of hospital rules, in the best interests of a patient (and perhaps against their own interests). If instead, we follow to the letter a set of rules even though we perceive them to be less than morally acceptable or appropriate to the specific context we are currently in, we are behaving in a deontological way, which is certainly less than moral, and which cannot really be defended morally, by claiming to have obeyed the rules. For a very public example of deontology, consider the behaviour of MPs over expenses. For a useful brief view on this and on deontology itself, see Longley (2010).

Teachers as educators

Teachers as educators of postgraduate professionals, by contrast to trainers, see themselves working with people who, as members of a profession, need to become rounded practitioners, and who need to be developed as *people* in terms of their knowing, doing, thinking, being and becoming.

To be a member of a profession — particularly one centred on work in a clinical setting — is inevitably to *be concerned with moral and ethical matters, and to seek the social good of one's clients/patients.* This in turn involves making professional judgements *on the spot,* in practice, rather than simply carrying out some pre-ordained activity without thinking about the particular instance involved. Thus, to *be able to make discretionary judgements is a characteristic of membership of a profession.* Professionals make such judgements by 'reading the situation', making meaning out of it and creating, at the time, a particular response to it based upon theoretical knowledge but also a range of other understandings, including sensitivity to the context. (See Fish and de Cossart 2007.) This requires the ability to think through the ethical and moral situation they are in and come to a conclusion that may not be traditionally orthodox. Such thinking is *not usually* regarded as something one can be trained to do. Rather, it requires a broad and in-depth education of the practitioner as a person, a professional and a knowledgeable and skilful doctor, through thoughtful discussion about specific cases.

The educational ends for which teachers as educators are responsible, are therefore to develop wise professionals (in this case, doctors), who can bring their whole person and character as well as their knowledge of themselves, their wider understanding, and their sound decision-making and wise professional judgement, to respond *appropriately* (and not automatically by protocol) to all the complexities, 'unpredictabilities' and particularities that their daily service to patients entails. Such medical teachers act as their own educational agent, choosing what is best for the given learner in the given context, by drawing on knowledge of the educational choices available, by analyzing the possibilities and opportunities found in the specific teaching context, and by being responsive to the learner's individual needs and interests as well as to the guidance of the learner's specialty college curriculum and its formal requirements. (The order here is significant in putting the individual learning doctor's needs first.)

Further, those educators who foster doctors' learning in clinical settings need to extend the learner's (and their own) criticality, and challenge what they take for granted in every aspect of their work. This should engage medical educators in considering sceptically their most cherished ideas, looking at the pros and cons of their decisions, and recognizing the costs and benefits.

The practice of education requires teachers who are already insightful and who demonstrate their own drawing together of critical perspectives and even their own uncertainties, as they teach. Such teachers facilitate learning and understanding, and ensure that this is underpinned by work set that ensures that learners make their own sense of what *they* know, do and think as they work. As we have seen, the educators' preparation for this is their own educational development. Thus the educator of educators has responsibilities that parallel those of teachers for their learners.

In the light of all this (which educators have known since Aristotle), it is embarrassing and ironic, that postgraduate doctors are still, in the 21st century, inaccurately referred to throughout the UK as 'trainees' and their clinical and educational supervisors are still known as trainers! The word 'training' implies that trainee's behaviour will be manipulated, whereas PGME is really about developing conduct.

Developing conduct, not changing behaviour

Where training changes behaviour, education is about developing conduct. *Behaviour* is used here to indicate a surface and visible set of actions and procedures that do not arise from inner conviction, but merely represent automatic activities that the trainer has inculcated in a learner (or are even outward acts that a learner has discerned as 'good to be seen doing', but which do not spring from personal conviction). Such training does not always produce long-term change, and is not owned by the trainee. *Conduct*, by contrast, here refers to learner's visible surface activities that are driven by their inner convictions, understandings, beliefs, values and character, which have been developed or shaped by education and which lie beneath that visible surface. The way people conduct themselves shows their true character (although anyone can do something that is 'out of character', and we use this phrase to indicate that it is not their normal conduct). A person's conduct is informed by the principles they believe in. It is about who they are, and as such characterizes them enduringly or until their understanding of what matters changes.

Other teaching roles and their inherent values, responsibilities and impact on learners

Before continuing with the main argument of this chapter, it is tempting here to review a range of other roles that teachers are sometimes labelled with, by choice or imposition, and to ask the simple question: what educational and other values underlie these roles, and, in what role do they cast the learner? Readers might also ask themselves in what role or roles they subconsciously see themselves, and whether 'playing a role' should be more than an occasional device for prompting learning. Consider, for example the following. Are there any roles listed in *Table 4.1 Some roles that teachers can adopt,* that are entirely inappropriate — in all circumstances — for a teacher to adopt?

Table 4.1 Some roles that teachers can adopt

Teacher as:			
	Entertainer	Dramatist	Presenter
	Instructor	Indoctrinator	Charismatic figure
	Moralist	Neutral chairman	Conversational partner
	Facilitator	Sounding board	Enabler
	Model	Inspiration	

As part of their planning for learning and as part of the judgements they make during a session, teachers need to think about the pros and cons of various ways of seeing themselves as teachers and of various roles that they might adopt. For example, a teacher might adopt a role as entertainer. But the usefulness of this crucially depends what this means. For example, although education should be fun, and an entertaining way of enabling learners to think about something carefully will be memorable and educationally worthwhile, to replace all education with mere 'edu-tainment' would arguably be to short-change learners. Thus, in seeking to be an entertainer, the good teacher has to maintain a careful balance that remains tilted towards the amusing only so long as it achieves educationally worthwhile ends. Further, given that sound education depends on a good relationship with the learner, it is important that learners understand who their teachers really are!

Similar dilemmas arise in respect of teacher as inspiration and/or charismatic figure. Here the teacher who is seduced into deliberately adopting these roles is arguably more interested in themselves than in their learners. This is because in such roles, while the teacher may be having an enjoyable time they may be reducing the learner's ability to think for themselves. The roles of instructor, presenter and indoctrinator may be inimical to achieving sound educational intentions especially where the learner ceases to take responsibility for learning — though any of these may be adopted in role-play in order to make educational points.

For teachers in PGME who understand well that their role is educational (which means offering educationally worthwhile opportunities to their learner) these matters are relatively easy to tease out. For them, the more complex issue is rather *how best to articulate the moral basis of their work.* In order to help readers construct their own reasoning about what it means to work in the moral mode of practice, the following is offered. It represents a carefully crafted argument by Hansen (2001) that demonstrates that teaching as a practice has its own integrity. It also shows that for those who are thoughtful about what they do as teachers for the sake of their learners and the ultimate protection and improvement of patient safety, teaching in PGME is already a moral and intellectual practice, and they are already part of its rich tradition.

Teaching as a moral activity: what it means to work in the moral mode of practice

As a practice, education's moral and intellectual terms and meanings *are derived from within us, as teachers.* Education need not be, as some think, an enterprise that is purely determined by political, social, economic or other interests and people with power outside and beyond our own arenas. Who we are, what we believe, what we value, and how we conduct ourselves as teachers, and how we relate to our learners is the real basis of teaching. This is why educators need to attend to their own character (personhood) and that of their learners, as well as to their understanding.

As we have seen, a focus on the *technical means* of teaching (the skills and strategies) — without considering the character of the learner or the personhood of the teacher, and the ends to which these are put — renders the activity of teaching sterile and turns it into:

▶ *a job* with clear-cut tasks which traditionally requires the transmission of knowledge, where telling the learner is enough

▶ *an occupation* where those outside it set the terms and conditions and the activities then have to be carried out as required, by an inside agent

▶ *a profession* offering specialized activities, but where we can still be diverted from thinking about the moral and the intellectual by other concerns like the paucity of time and resources.

Equally, to focus instead only on *the ends,* can lead to 'outcomes-focused' approaches, where the product is: socializing; acculturating; producing productive members of society; shaping successful and compliant workers. This would take us back to training.

Instead, Hansen argues, teachers, 'should first determine what they care about, and then craft a conception of teaching that coheres with that determination' (Hansen 2001: 4). For example in PGME, it would be reassuring for patients to know that medical educators think about how their learner is developing as a person, care about what kind of a doctor their learner will become, are concerned about how their learners will conduct themselves at the bedside. Such teachers might also care about how well their learner thinks, how well they make decisions, and how wise their judgements are becoming. Such matters might need to embellish the national requirements in respect of what the doctor needs to learn.

This, of course, is another way of saying that educators of professionals need to have examined carefully their professional moral values as teachers and also the values of the profession in which they are working with learners. Such values will then enable them to develop educational aims with which they are comfortable and which attend to their learners' needs as discovered in studying those learners. These ideas should be used to enable the teacher to become their own agent, attending to the requirements of the curriculum, but also beyond that to the deeper and undocumented but important needs of their learners. Indeed, in PGME, as in all education for postgraduate practice, this will also enable teachers to support learners in considering and expressing their own philosophy of practice and in recognizing how this relates to that of their profession more generally and the quality of the practice they engage in.

None of this, of course, is new. But it is something which seems to have evaporated in the rush and tumble, the white noise and the urgency, that currently characterize medical practice in an NHS that seems to focus more on business than on care, more on economies and targets than on the real reason it is there. Refocusing on and re-enlivening the moral traditions of medicine and education might rebalance the scales.

As Hansen points out, a moral tradition has animated teaching ever since the days of Socrates and Confucius. And there are huge parallels here for medical practice also. In education, this tradition has enabled a dialogue about teaching and education to take place across the generations. In that dialogue the encounter with the past is what helps us to curb the instrumentalist tendencies of the present (which endlessly try to encroach on our consciousness as important in today's busy world). The best of educational traditions can be safeguarded when the practice of teaching (as handed down through time), does not constitute a hardened and unchangeable endeavour to which teachers must bind themselves, but rather is a living practice which evolves as a result of the initiative and imagination of teachers whose very task is to respond *thinkingly* to current external pressures and social demands in the light of their beliefs and understandings about their profession's practice (see Hansen 2001:9).

Thus, teaching is a living practice that is nurtured by tradition (though some of its practices have blossomed and then withered, over several cycles). And it is a practice that has endured for a very long time by maintaining its core identity and continuity even as it develops. Some teachers may be leaders who shape this role. They give it intellectual and moral substance, and their best ideas are enshrined in some of the most important literature on teaching (which is why teachers need to be aware of it so as to access and learn from it). But such writers are also echoing the components of teaching that have developed over time.

Some of the enduring traditions of good teaching include: enabling students to think in broader rather than narrower terms; fuelling (rather than draining) learners' confidence; deepening, rather than weakening learners' engagement with the larger world they inhabit. The following is highlighted as being four of the most important paragraphs in this book.

Morally sound teachers give sustained intellectual and moral attention to their learners. They study them. They are *intellectually attentive* to them by focusing on what these learners know, can do, feel and think. They are *morally attentive* to them by being alert to their learners' responses to opportunities to *grow as persons* (to become more rather than less thoughtful about ideas, and more rather than less sensitive to others' views and concerns). They are mindful that every learner is unique, with a distinctive set of dispositions, capabilities, understandings and outlooks. Thus the bonds between teacher and learner are intellectual and moral, pertaining to their emerging knowledge, understanding and growth as persons. (See Hansen 2001.)

Further, the motivation of such teachers is a crucial component in their moral practice. They conduct themselves as described above, not as a means to an end, but because that is what they see as 'being a teacher'. Indeed, as Hansen argues, to seek to become a good teacher is a calling or vocation, felt within the practitioner, and which cannot be achieved by extrinsic obligation. Though, I would argue, it might be nudged into life by increasing intellectual understanding of the nature of education and the growth of the practitioner as a person who learns what it is to see and think as a teacher.

Teaching is particularly about interacting educationally with a learner. Clearly, the person the teacher is has a considerable bearing on how they interact with (and even what they achieve with) learners. Thus the concept 'person' is central to the practice of teaching. Usefully, by the same token, this is also true of the doctor who (as we argued in Fish and de Cossart 2007, chapter nine) needs to bring their whole person to meet the whole person the patient is. The idea of 'conduct' here helps to capture the intellectual and moral presence a teacher develops. Learners learn as much from a teacher's conduct as from the subject they teach!

The moral sensibility and the moral authority of the teacher (summed up in the qualities of the *person* that they bring to bear in their teaching) are the most influential factors in achieving fruitful learning. This requires the teacher to bring to the encounter understanding, knowledge, initiative and receptivity. (See Hansen 2001:20.) Such a teacher will have a sense of educational agency, will be able to articulate *properly educational* aims, and act on them, will think about what they do as they are doing it, will be able to make wise judgements and choose the best teaching strategies on behalf of the learner both during preparation and in the midst of the action, will hold learners in positive regard, will sometimes have personal feelings towards them, but will also have insight into their strengths and weaknesses and will be able to take a disinterested interest in them. In short, they will put the learner and the learner's welfare first in their thinking.

So, in the light of this, what is 'good' teaching?

Many learners will take a 'good' teacher for granted, as if teachers naturally have inherent 'teacherly' qualities. This is commonly referred to in the statement that a good teacher is born and not made. To some extent this is true, since many of the important qualities on which good teaching rests are, for many, innate. However, as Carr, D. (2007) shows, there is a difference here between character, which can be developed, and personality, which may be less susceptible to development. This notion of innate teacherly qualities therefore underrates the number of components that a teacher must work at, and the amount of work they need to put in over the years, in order to teach well. And many of these qualities and components are indeed able to be learnt or developed, and have been developed, through hard work, by many people. So what then can we say about the good teacher?

It should be noted that the argument in this section is informed by the work of David Carr (See Carr, D. 2004) and Palmer (1998). Carr explains that to label something 'good', is to indicate that it is a *virtue in itself* — that it is an end in itself, that it is the realization of a transcendent 'good' (which means you do it for its own sake, not for an ulterior motive)! Good teaching, then, is a virtue in itself.

When attached to the word 'teaching', it also indicates that 'good' is the goal for the practice of teaching. That is: 'Good' teaching is a means to 'good ends', in that it enables learners to gain valuable and worthwhile things — like understanding and knowledge.

Carr notes that the current vogue in teacher education generally is for competency-based teaching. This requires teachers 'who are in training to enter the profession', to make observable in their teaching practice several hundred competencies — referred to in some documents as *repertoires of definable operationisable skills*. There is a very large list of these, and 'good teaching' is currently standardized against this list. Thus, in this view, 'good teaching' by definition means having a specified number of competencies or 'skills'.

Carr also makes articulate an important rebuttal of this approach. He argues that the degree to which it is *good* teaching depends rather: 'on the possession and exercise by the teacher of a range of virtues of a broadly Aristotelian kind, including practical wisdom (*phronesis*)'. He also argues that we as teachers should not be embarrassed to acknowledge (recognize overtly) how much the Aristotelian (and the Thomist) virtues *are embodied in the character, rather than in the technical proficiency* of a good teacher. (The Thomist virtues, refers to the Christian values that Thomas Aquinas articulated in the 13th Century in his *Summa Theologica*.) For a list of both Aristotelian and Thomist virtues, see The Appendix, p.205.

Carr further makes it clear that a good teacher is good more because s/he is a good person than because s/he possesses 'X' number of organizational skills and teaching strategies. As he points out, great teachers of the past were 'great persons' who taught! I would add to this by arguing that those whom we personally saw as 'bad teachers' are almost always those somewhat lacking in some qualities of character that make for good interaction with learners, although some also lacked a structured knowledge of their subject.

Further, as we have shown, good teaching is not really so much about good performance (being drilled in skills, measured for the observable, and conforming to rules laid down by an outside agent). Rather, it is more about the teacher's character, that drives a moral awareness and a moral mode of engagement with learners such that the teacher is an agent of their own teaching (choosing the what, why and the how of their work) — guided, but not constrained, by the curriculum, and able to use discretion (professional judgement) in the light of the context.

Palmer (1998) writes about the inner character of the good teacher in very different and rather more poetic but equally important ways. He builds his book on the simple premise that: 'good teaching cannot be reduced to technique; good teaching comes from the identity and integrity of the teacher' (Palmer 1998: 10). He then later adds:

If identity and integrity are more fundamental to good teaching than technique — ... we must do something alien to academic culture: we must talk to each other about our inner lives — risky stuff in a profession that fears the personal and seeks safety in the technical.

(ibid: 12)

He defines identity as 'an evolving nexus where all the forces that constitute my life converge in the mystery of self', and of integrity he says, 'I mean whatever wholeness I am able to find within that nexus as its vectors form and reform the pattern of my life'. (Ibid: 13).

Of the teacher's authority he says, tellingly, 'Authority is granted to people who are perceived as authoring their own words, their own actions, their own lives, rather than playing a scripted role at a great remove from our own hearts'. He adds: 'Authority comes as I reclaim my identity and integrity ... then teaching comes from the depths of my own truth' (Palmer 1998: 33). This resonates strongly with the issues raised in chapter two about the teacher being their own agent. The key intention of such educators is to improve the learner's understanding (by discussing with them a wider range of possible ways of thinking) such that this changed understanding will change practice for the better.

Palmer's interest is particularly in 'the courage to teach' and he makes the important point that 'what we teach will never "take" unless it connects with the inward, living core of our students' lives'. This, he shows, requires teachers to have explored and reflected in depth on their own practice and on what they bring to it. He says: 'when we have not sounded our own depths, we cannot sound the depths of our students' lives', (Palmer 1998: 31).

By comparison with David Carr's very helpful philosophical points earlier, Palmer's words may seem less scholarly. But readers who feel that this more person-focused approach is less than credible as a subject for postgraduate doctors, are referred back to the consultant's words in the box at the front of this chapter.

Thus, seeking to become a good teacher is about recognizing the inextinguishably moral dimension of teaching and understanding why, in seeking to become a good teacher, one is called to personal transformation of heart and soul. It also means that for teachers and their learners it is important to attend to the rationales and debates about medicine and education *as practices*. This requires of medical educators that, as a base level, they should be supported nationally to climb the mountain of educational practice at least as far as beginning to think like a teacher.

This brings us to the final responsibility of the teacher, which is to reflect upon and learn from their teaching in order to develop it further and/or improve it. As a basis for this, teachers need to engage in a proper process of evaluation. In the technical mode of practice this is achieved through a simple tick list (sometimes with a Likert scale), and asks narrow and pre-formulated questions of learners, immediately at the end of the session. In the moral mode of practice, evaluation would be construed as follows.

Evaluating teaching

At the heart of the term 'evaluation' lies the word 'value'. The evaluation of an *educational* enterprise should thus be concerned with exploring and reflecting on:

▷ the intentions and the value of the education offered

▷ the quality of the ideas and experiences, and the support offered to the learner

▷ the soundness of the principles that lay beneath the education provided

▷ what it has altered or developed in the learner — if at all yet.

This is not the same as asking whether learners have enjoyed it, found it 'comfortable', or how they rated, or even recognized, the teacher's skills. The role of education is to challenge, to enable learners to 'see anew', and gain new insights. (This may be less than totally comfortable at the time, and may even make some people grumpy!) This is why evaluations that declare unalloyed pleasure in the teaching provided, and complete comfort with the content and processes, merely show that the learner has not been challenged and probably that the teacher has not done the job! It is also why one-off evaluation sheets, filled in immediately the session ends, will never do justice to what has been learnt, because the enlightenment that education affords often develops slowly in the learner, such that what they felt was unhelpful on the occasion can prove to have been invaluable in the light of later understanding and hindsight. Thus, while training cashes out into immediate and visible changes (of behaviour), education, which changes *understanding*, takes longer to show and its true value for an individual learner may be fully recognized only much later.

Educational evaluation seeks to investigate and understand the processes that have taken place in an educational enterprise, with a view to developing or refining them. It is to be distinguished from *assessment* (which is concerned with student progress)

and *appraisal* (which is concerned with staff "performance" as seen by the employer).

The worth of education does not readily yield to simple visible and measurable outcomes. It is a 'category mistake' to seek to quantify something that cannot be measured!

Educational evaluation is a form of educational research and particularly of practitioner enquiry. The processes and intentions of such enquiries need to take account of the nature of professional practice itself, which should shape the collection of evidence, and its interpretation. Such research requires the exploration of multiple perspectives because, being about complex human issues which are three-dimensional, it needs to be studied from at least three perspectives in order to do it full justice. Thus using for 'the evaluation' *only* a questionnaire filled in by learners on the day is not good enough.

Current rhetoric requires educational evaluation to be dressed in the guise of Quality Assurance. However, it should never be forgotten that the best way of guaranteeing the quality of professional practice is not an elaborate administrative superstructure, but rather a process which supports critical enquiry, deepening understanding, and consequent review and development of the educational processes at work in teaching and learning. It should also be remembered that, as Onora O'Neill says:

> Plants don't flourish when we pull them up too often to check how their roots are growing: political, institutional and professional life too may not flourish if we constantly uproot it to demonstrate that everything is transparent and trustworthy.
>
> *(O'Neill 2002: 19)*

Such review and development needs to relate to the educational aims of the teacher as well as the means and the outcomes. Traditionally, teachers find articulating their educational aims and intentions or objectives particularly hard. But such aims are the inescapable starting point for successful teaching. The following chapter therefore seeks to help with this. Further help in designing teaching either in major programmes or even as self-standing sessions can be found in Fish and Coles (2005).

Further reading

* Hansen, D. (2001) *Exploring the Moral Heart of Teaching.* London: Teachers College Press (Preface and chapter two).

* Palmer, Parker J. (1998) *The Courage to Teach.* San Francisco: Jossey Bass (chapter one).

Chapter Five

Seeing the overall purpose anew: starting from aims and intentions that are properly educational

> Asking a person about his [sic] aims is a method of getting him to concentrate or clear his mind about what he is trying to achieve. 'Aim' also carries the suggestion that we are trying to achieve something that we might fall short of because of the difficulty involved in the task. ... To ask questions about the aims of education is therefore a way of getting people to get clear about and focus their attention on what is worthwhile achieving. ... Whatever he says he is aiming at, the formulation of his aim is an aid in making his activity more structured and coherent by isolating an aspect under which he is acting. It [formulating educational aims] is not something which he does in order to explain what he is doing, it is rather, a more precise specification of it [of what he is doing].
>
> *(Peters 1966: 28-29)*
>
> ... in formulating aims of education we are attempting to specify more precisely what qualities ... we think it most desirable to develop.
>
> *(Hirst and Peters 1970:16)*

Introduction
An overview of the logic of educational aims and intentions
Some key issues about educational aims
Aims arising from the nature of education
Further reading

Introduction

For those senior clinicians whose teaching I observed before they joined their PG Cert, formulating the *educational* aims of a session proved to be the least well attended to aspect of preparing for their enterprise. Further, only one made any attempt to link what they did with learners to the aims of their learner's formal curriculum, and the broad goals of postgraduate medical education were left tacit. Some did make descriptive statements about what they were going to *do* in their session (operational aims) or even how they were going to 'manage' the session (managerial aims). But no-one, at that point, could articulate any wider view of the nature of education. Thus they had no basis from which to construct any educational aims, based upon *what it is to educate* and focused on *the kind of doctor they were ultimately trying to cultivate.*

Many books have been written, on both sides of the Atlantic, on the subject of the aims of education, but these focus on the aims of school education and /or are more concerned with a philosophical enquiry into the complexity of articulating sound and logical aims that can be agreed broadly. (See, for example: Whitehead (1932); Peters

(1966); Hirst and Peters (1970); Brown (1970); White (1982); and the very useful collection edited by Roger Marples (1999/2002). However, apart from Fish and Coles (2005) chapter four, there seems to be little written on the aims of postgraduate medical education and how teachers in clinical practice can use them as the basis for formulating the kind of postgraduate doctor they are seeking to develop. Amongst many of the above writers, there is, however, broad agreement about the need to 'ground' educational aims (longer term goals) in a clearly delineated conception of education itself (see, for example, Barrow 2002; Carr, D. 2002). This is about having a wider *educational view* of what it is to educate. Since we have already developed that view in earlier chapters (by delineating two modes of practice), we shall now explore the influence of each mode of practice on the expression of aims, and note that the more immediate means to these aims are usually summarized under the heading of 'objectives' within the technical mode of practice and under the term 'intentions' within the moral mode.

In the technical mode of practice, the activities engaged in by the trainer as teacher, with the trainee as learner, are instrumental (arise almost exclusively from the basic activities demanded by the job) and have been chosen, designed and required of them by some authority beyond them, which they must simply obey. The vocabulary most associated with training uses the term 'aims' (which is common across all planning for teaching) and also 'objectives'. For pure training these are 'behavioural objectives' which must be cast in visible and measurable terms (for example, by the end of the session the learner will be able to do a specific new action) or 'learning outcomes' (which state what the learner will have learnt by the end). The problem with this is that it is based on the assumption that all learning can be pre-planned and foretold, which removes the creativity from the interaction between teacher and learner, and makes the process unproductive for both.

For those who see themselves as working within the moral mode of practice, none of this seems likely to help shape educationally worthwhile experiences that will motivate either teacher or learners. For them, 'intentions' involves designing their learner's education so as to use their time as educationally as possible, by having a clear view of the main educational achievements that can and should arise from the session and setting up activities in which other, unexpected, educational benefits may also occur and prove seriously enlightening, on the day.

Very few of those observed, not having formulated their educational aims, were able to convey to their learners any detailed sense of what they sought to achieve with them. Rather, the teachers' thinking about their educational responsibilities seemed to start at a point *beyond* all this, and caused most of them to jump straight into the 'meat of the session', on the basis of unstated assumptions about its intentions, direction and structure (and of course these assumptions were not automatically shared by the learner). Beneath all this lies a tacit, even naïve, assumption that everyone knows what education for postgraduate doctors is all about, and that it is incontestable and straightforward. Indeed, probably most of those I saw had simply never been made aware of the importance of formulating educational aims. Further, this may well be true of the majority of their colleagues.

To chase the real responsibility of this back to its roots, it seems fair to recognize that a consensus of the overall educational aims of PGME has never been writ large anywhere, and that a public debate about them is long overdue. Further, few national medical curricula start by making either general or specialty-focused statements about their educational aims talking instead about preparing doctors for the next stage of their career, or for a role as consultant.

This seems to be an amazing — even horrifying — state of affairs for medicine and for healthcare in the United Kingdom — unless, of course you do not believe that educational aims matter. And this comes back to one's educational values. In the technical mode of practice, it is probably clear (though tacit) at all levels, that PGME is about 'making' the trainee conform to the specific knowledge and skill required at work and laid down in the syllabus of the curriculum, and that the teacher's role is to tell, instruct and test a learner who in return will listen, do as required and demonstrate through set assessment procedures their newly acquired competencies. The kind of learner (postgraduate doctor) that this approach results in (as an obedient, passive and uncritical receiver of training and jumper of hurdles), is itself very worrying. In the moral mode of practice, however, as this chapter will show, it is part of the responsibility of the teacher to have thought through and formulated their educational aims and intentions for all their teaching, such that their time with the learner is clearly educationally focused.

This chapter seeks to support the wider debate about the educational aims of PGME, which this book as a whole is promoting. It also provides for the more immediate needs of teachers to set appropriate aims for their teaching on the ground (both to set a direction for their entire programme and to guide the careful expression of the intentions of their individual sessions). In building on earlier chapters, this chapter offers in three main sections a range of perspectives on educational aims for the education of postgraduate doctors. These are as follows: (i) an overview of the logic of educational aims; (ii) some key issues about educational aims (iii) aims arising from the nature of education as an enterprise.

An overview of the logic of educational aims and intentions

Educational aims are best constructed by considering firstly the nature of the overall educational enterprise that they will characterize. For teachers of postgraduate doctors, this means beginning from the wider view, held perhaps nationally, of how the nature of practice of medicine should be construed now and for the future, and therefore how we might characterize the nature of medical education. This then also requires consideration and critique by each teacher, of what medicine as a practice does and should involve, and the formulation of a personal philosophy that provides their starting point for more detailed planning. The resulting statement of aims will then resonate both with the overall aims of PGME, as the profession's view, and with the individual's own educational philosophy. However, this enterprise is jeopardized at the start because finding a clear statement about the overall *educational aims* of postgraduate medical education in any of the documentation of the GMC, PMETB, The British Medical Association (BMA), or even AoME, seems impossible, and none of the Royal Colleges' curricula start from here either.

The bodies that oversee PGME (the GMC, the BMA and AoME) all have aims *for themselves as public bodies*, but the phrase 'educational aims of postgraduate medicine' does not seem to appear in any literature. Even PMETB in its statement of *The principles of good medical education and training* (now taken over by the GMC) speaks of education as being about doctors acquiring 'the knowledge, skills, attitudes and behaviours necessary to keep up to date' (principle 52) and: all 'education and training should be based on the need to promote health care that focuses on patients and shared decision-making (principle 48). Not even the Gold Guide to specialty training mentions 'educational aims', and the aims it does discuss are managerial ones. That is why this book calls for a debate about the aims of PGME. An example of such overall aims is therefore offered, as follows, in *Frame 5.1 Possible aims for Postgraduate Medical Education*.

Frame 5.1 Possible aims for Postgraduate Medical Education

> Postgraduate Medical Education should seek to nurture and develop a doctor who is wise in judgement, sound in decision-making, aware of their professional responsibilities, appropriately knowledgeable and skilful, keen to continue their professional development, of a lively and flexible mind, who shows sensitivity to others, has criticality and is capable of being pro-active in the interests of justice and fairness for the patient's well-being. Such a doctor can bring all these attributes, united within the whole person they are, to the service of the patient, whom they will meet without undue self-interest (except for the need to attend to their own basic health and wellbeing), and for whom they care, beyond the protocol-driven spirit of 'delivering' care packages and pathways.
>
> A simpler version might speak of cultivating the character and personal qualities of the learning doctor alongside the knowledge, skills, and capacities appropriate for a professional whose calling is to serve patients and seek the greater health of the nation.
>
> Another view is that: 'the aim of medical education is to develop medical expertise that consists of intuition and metacognition'. (Quirk 2006:125)

It is irrefutable that such aims are inspirational and idealist. But without such a vision, how can educators know what they are trying to achieve (and whether or not they have achieved it)? As Peters says (quoted in the box at the start of the chapter): 'The word "Aim" also carries the suggestion that we are trying to achieve something that we might fall short of because of the difficulty involved in the task'.

How do educational aims, ends or goals relate to educational intentions?

There is a proper logic that relates overall long-term educational aims to the aims of a specific programme, which in turn shapes the specific educational intentions for a given teaching interaction within that programme. Currently PGME is clearly not aware of, and thus does not attend to, this logic.

The problem is as follows.

1. Since the overall long-term educational aims for the whole of PGME have not been agreed and made explicit through national debate, these long-term aims exist only tacitly. Thus, where PGME might be construed as an enterprise that seeks to educate doctors in specific values, virtues, conduct, judgement and character as well as in terms of their necessary knowledge and skill, the current tacit aim is no more specific than seeking to create a consultant capable of working in a particular specialty as a result of previous successful experience in a range of foundation and specialty-related areas.

2. Since the specialty curricula also do not make the educational aims for their programme explicit, the education offered within a department (which should emerge from the overall aims) is probably tacitly construed as 'to pass the attachment successfully and fulfil the syllabus requirements'.

3. This in turn means that the learning agreement, on the basis of which the teacher and the learner negotiate what that learner's whole programme for the attachment will seek to achieve, provides a very indeterminate basis for such negotiation — beyond listing the syllabus to be covered.

4. It is not, therefore surprising that the short-term intentions for individual teaching sessions in PGME (which should be derived from the learning agreement and relate directly to its aims) are not given educational shape and point, and often slip into attending only to the explicit items listed in the syllabus — which all relate to skills and knowledge.

In fact, both long-term aims and short-term intentions need to be considered together by the teacher, in order to ensure that our short-term intentions do not compromise our longer-term aims. For example, setting out to tell the learner speedily what to do in a given situation may produce some immediate results that are pleasing, but in the longer term may make the learner dependent on the teacher and uncritically accepting of whatever authority directs, when the longer-term aims are to nurture criticality and independence.

Aims, goals and ends

The overall educational achievements to be sought within PGME generally, and specialty programmes in particular, and within which teacher and learner work, can be referred to by three nouns: 'aims'; 'ends' and 'goals', which can be used interchangeably in relation to the adjective 'educational'. But they do have slightly different nuances. The word 'aims' is most commonly used in formal educational planning and indicates aspirations. Both the terms 'goals' and 'ends' have more of an instrumental thrust, perhaps suggesting that the end product is more important than the processes used to achieve it, which in turn could result in a choice of means to such goals that are less than moral. The word 'ends' is sometimes used by philosophers to highlight the idea that an educator is working towards ideals that may be less than totally definable.

Planning your aims and intentions as a teacher

In preparing for their educational activities with their individual learner on the ground, teachers should bring together a view of what might be the wider aims of PGME, clarify their own more detailed aims (for their whole programme) and use these to shape the intentions in the individual session, ensuring that these are all compatible. It should be noted that where they have the choice, their expression of aims and intentions is always shaped by the educator's own underlying values. These need to be transparent because the educator is inevitably promoting them through both their choice of focus and also through the words in which these are expressed. Intentions emerge from studying the learner, what they currently understand and can do, their needs and interests, as well as taking proper account of the formal curriculum the learner is following. Educational intentions for teaching in the clinical setting are about what the teacher is trying to achieve educationally within the immediate activities of their teaching.

Thus, educational intentions for any given session needs to be considered and expressed in relation to the curriculum and the departmental programme which that learner is following. Such intentions need to be shaped by what is achievable in the one session. They come first in a teacher's thinking about what, when, how, why and where to teach *this learner*. Logically, (if the enterprise is to be counted as education) the teacher's intentions must be about what is educationally worthwhile for this learner on this occasion, and must consider this before all other decisions about how to teach, learn, assess, and evaluate the educational experience. All other decisions about teaching, learning and assessment then should follow logically from these intentions.

Some key issues about educational aims

In relating intentions back to educational aims, teachers in PGME will find themselves considering a number of wider issues. This is a less onerous task if shared with colleagues. Indeed, a number of voices here will enrich these important debates. This section seeks to explore some of these issues.

When educational terms are discussed, conflicting views are often expressed, because education is values-based and therefore its ideas are contestable. As Standish (1999) points out long-term educational aims are located in three areas: the needs of society; the need to 'pass on and develop those ways of knowing and understanding which are the common heritage'; and the need to attend to 'a process of unfolding from within [the learner] or through an authentic creation [or re-creation] of themselves.

All these have something to say to medical educators. The first reminds us that society (every aspect from politicians and the media, to patients and their relatives) has a stake in the PGME enterprise. The second reminds us that there is in teachers and current practice much wisdom and experience as well as knowledge and skill, which learners deserve to explore (rather than simply absorb). The third reminds us of the importance of developing the individual doctor's whole being as the person who meets and cares for the patient. (See Standish 1999: 35-6.)

This is why a fair and open debate needs to be conducted about the balance of these aims, within medical and surgical departments and the wider faculty of teachers within a single Health Care Provider. Views need to be aired and then in order to make progress there has to be democratic agreement based on a common consensus about the most important issues. This section seeks to consider some of the more difficult issues that can muddy the waters of debate. As White (1982) has shown these include the following.

▷ Do we need aims at all, and if so, who should determine them and what should be considered in framing them?

▷ Why should teachers not simply leave their educational ends to others at a higher level and only concern themselves with the means to those ends?

▷ Aren't learners' abilities and achievements determined by what nature has endowed them with, in which case, what can education do?

▷ Should the teacher of professionals be concerned with the learners' personal qualities and dispositions, values and character, and if so how?

Do we need aims at all, and if so, who should determine them and what should be considered in framing them?

Education is surely an intentional and purposeful enterprise. Without a clear sense of where they are trying to go, neither medical teacher nor learning doctor can be sure what they have achieved, how educationally valuable that was, and how well it related to the learner's professional needs. This seems a fairly persuasive case for sound education needing to be based on educational aims. The case is made above (pp. 35-7) for teachers to be their own agents, and to own the aims by which they work (which may be through considered agreement with those designed by higher authority and/or by additionally articulating their own).

Thus, clear aims for the *programme* that the learner is on in the given attachment need to be agreed by all from whom the 'trainee' will learn. This will certainly be more than their clinical and educational supervisor, because everyone the learner meets will have an educational influence, directly or indirectly. The aims of the departmental programme (like the rest of the programme) may well be an amalgam of the learner's formal curriculum (if it contains aims) and what the particular department believes is necessary for a learner in this specialty to achieve educationally, as well as what the department can offer. The programme's aims provide the rationality for the smaller-scale intentions of any teaching. These in turn will shape and determine the what, when and how of the specific teaching and learning processes.

However, it should also be remembered that for teachers to (have to) set out with a very narrow set of intentions, from which they will not deviate, will deprive teachers and learners alike of the creative adventure that education can and should also be. Like many of these matters, a careful balance needs to be kept between the pre-determined agenda and the impromptu opportunities that arise in a session. Having formulated their educational intentions for a session, the teacher is in a better position to achieve this balance by being flexible to follow useful ideas from the learner and making sound educational judgements about this, even as they teach. Thus, it is clear that it is the teacher who must take final responsibility for formulating the educational thrust of their teaching. This is a serious and significant responsibility.

Why should we as educators be concerned with educational ends and not simply the means?

One suggestion often made is that education should be concerned solely with *means* (the ways of teacher engaging with learners and how they learn, including what assessment can tell us), so that we can leave those at a higher level to tell us what education should consist of and what teachers therefore should seek to achieve. The contrasting view of course is that leaving others outside education to determine educational aims is to lay open the educational enterprise to political interference, to the possible corruption of the whole process, and to aims that are far from educational.

The argument that a teacher should contribute also to the design of the broad educational aims of a curriculum is worth considering, but it will only stand up so long as educators attend properly to a range of views and documents, motives and interests from an appropriate range of those with a legitimate stake in the learners' education. This is why (as made clear in Fish and Coles, 2005), it is important for the formal curriculum to be debated by an appropriate range of contributors. It is also vital for individual teachers in shaping their work to recognize their accountability to patients, learners, and the whole faculty of teaching colleagues, in addition to being sensitive to the demands of the formal curriculum, the needs and interests of the learner and the context of the learning, including changing societal views. Under these mitigating influences, it would also then be seen as acceptable for the teacher to use their authority to promote certain educationally worthwhile ends.

Aren't learners' abilities and achievements determined by what nature has endowed them with, in which case what can education do?

If education is 'upbringing', then how should we bring up learning doctors? What achievements of character, intellect, skill, knowledge do we and they have in mind as legitimate educational goals? Or are learners' abilities and character innate and not a proper subject for education? This is also an issue to be faced in determining educational aims — even for postgraduate doctors.

These questions raise what educators know as the 'nature/nurture debate', because there are two ways of looking at what learners bring to their education and can gain from education, and these affect what an educator's aims should and can be.

The biological model of education has nature at its core and its key metaphor is 'growth'. This view has been attributed to progressive educationists who believe that education is a process of growth or development towards a final end, and that that final end is the cultivation of individuality, self-realization, and the fullest development of one's potential. Here, the teacher stands back and encourages 'flowering'. However, overdone, this can be so learner-centred that teachers can appear to make no interventions at all. This is what happened to progressive education when a few primary schools in the 1970s were shown to be failing to intervene properly in the children's activities so that very little education was apparently taking place, and suddenly all progressive education was then deemed to be a failure.

The social model of education holds that nurture is the core of true education. Here the prevailing metaphor is initiation. Here, education is a social enterprise during which rules that are agreed as the product of a society must be learnt. 'Traditional education' was (and is) the term for this. Here the teacher is an intermediary between society and the child, and culture and the child, and must deliberately intervene in learning to initiate the learner into public rules, publicly valued knowledge, and the cultural modes of society. However, overdone, this can lead to subtle indoctrination of the set of values of one society, or class or group.

Of course, both these views of what education should be about contain useful ideas for a teacher trying to formulate sound educational aims. The following section considers some of this in terms of medical education.

Should the teacher of professionals be concerned with the learners' personal qualities and dispositions, values and character, and if so how?

In examining the practice of doctors we can see that, as Carr, D. says of teachers, 'their effectiveness is greatly enhanced by the possession and exercise of personal qualities and practical dispositions that are not entirely (if at all) reducible to academic knowledge or technical skills' (Carr, D. 2007: 369). Indeed, patients respond to doctors in the light of who they are as people and what they deduce of their needs and values by watching and listening to them. Seen within the moral mode of practice, the personal qualities, values and character that the doctor brings to meet the patient, are endemic to the quality of their professional practice as a whole.

What we might speak of here as inherent in good medical practice are appropriate personal qualities, professional values, and character. Clearly, following the lead of Carr (2007) we could argue that a whole range of personal qualities and dispositions are important for medical practice. These surely include the GMC list that describes the Good Doctor, but this offers a very conservative mix of items that no one from any cultural background would disagree with. By contrast, the list of Aristotelian and Thomist virtues (see Appendix) might well serve as a starting point for key qualities of character. If these matter, and if they can be developed (both of which this book argues for), then these should be part of our educational aims and indeed, may be seen as 'permeating themes' in all our teaching. Then we would have a virtues-based curriculum instead of a competencies-based one!

This also raises some other issues in respect of the medical educator's responsibilities regarding the learner's personality and character. For example: can these things be taught? Arguably, they can — at least by both modelling good conduct and by open and direct discussion of the very points raised here. Shouldn't the differences in learners also be fostered, alongside some requirements for conformity? Arguably they should, and finding the right balance for this — for each individual learner — is an important ability in a PGME teacher. Further, given that learner-centred intentions cannot be the sole aims of education, how should they be related to other educational aims? Again, arguably, this is about keeping a balance between all the educator's responsibilities to the learner. A few second's thought will suggest that although these are difficult responsibilities for the teacher, they will be greatly helped by having carefully formulated appropriate educational intentions beforehand, for that learner. This itself is part of the important professional judgements that teachers make in preparing to teach. Thus, the educator's job is both to enlighten the learner's understanding (to be able to know enough to make sound choices) and to be self-aware enough to be able to develop character, personal qualities and dispositions. The teacher cannot escape being responsible for the twin aims of helping the learner to possess knowledge and understanding, and to develop the necessary dispositions to use this wisely — because the educated learner can't have one without the other!

For many (if not most) educators this will include developing moral dispositions, which will be a particularly important aim for the teacher of postgraduate doctors. Learning doctors whose moral dispositions have been well developed, means that they:

▷ have a theoretical understanding of their profession's ethical rules and moral principles

▷ are inclined (through habituation) to follow these rules and principles (have been led to form, develop or become a morally virtuous character)

▷ actually have moral virtues as part of their character.

This is about 'bringing up' a learner to be able to apply, and *actually to apply*, their moral understanding to virtuous ends, (otherwise, it is possible to use moral knowledge for wicked ends, or to be too weak to do what is known to be 'the right thing').

In seeking to develop moral dispositions, many compromises may be necessary! For example: learner-centred intentions (that which is designed for the good of the learner and attends to their wants or needs or interests) will have to be balanced by socially- and societally-focused aims, and wider professional ones. Another example is that self-individualization needs to be balanced by moral awareness and commitment to moral actions that go beyond and may conflict with the ethics of society or one's profession. Indeed, the individual good and the common good may not coincide. So should a doctor in a practice situation: settle for a trimmed down version of morality; or consciously and temporally separate them; or deliberately or unconsciously disconnect their own motives and attitudes from what they are required to do; or sacrifice themselves for the common good? Arguably, we need to bring up the learner to understand these complexities, to find their way through them, and even to see that a benevolent person is more likely to live a good life than an egoist! If so, then these are also educational aims that an educator will need to express beyond those agreed nationally, and in expressing them, they may find that they have sharpened their own understandings of them, thus becoming better prepared to educate learners about them.

In addition to these matters, the nature of education and how we construe it will also influence the way we articulate our aims.

Aims arising from the nature of education

Once the teacher seeks to be an educator, they are on the way to considering what 'to act educationally' means. This involves recognizing that education lies in the moral mode of practice, with all that follows from this for the teacher, in terms of pursuing educationally worthwhile ends and seeking to realize worthwhile virtues. This can be summed up by saying that educational practice is: 'morally informed and morally committed action', in which the educator enables the processes of growth in the learner. (See Carr, W. 1995: 64 and 68). It is emancipatory and liberating for the individual and is the practice of freedom in which learners discover themselves and achieve their humanity (see Fish and Coles (2005).

The arguments are as follows in the following four key points and commentary.

1. A practice cannot be claimed as educational unless it is underpinned by (implicit or explicit) understanding of what it is 'to act educationally'.

It is broadly agreed by educators that to act educationally is to open minds, liberate thinking, encourage critique, explore the foundations of good practice and develop creativity, as well as to involve learners in intrinsic motivation by using their interests as a vehicle for what needs to be learnt. (See as key authors the work of: Oakeshott, M.; Carr, D.; Carr, W.; Dewey, J.; Freire, P.; Palmer, P.J.; Van Manen, M.; Wilson, P.S.)

Commentary

It is important to note that where activity engaged in is 'educational' (does open minds, liberate thinking, encourage critique and so on), teachers may, *irrespective of their teacherly 'know-how' or skills, claim to practise in an educational way*, (see Carr, W. 1995: 160). But where the activity chosen by the teacher is not genuinely educational, or educationally worthwhile, *no amount of cleverly performed or up-to-date teaching skills will compensate,* and no technical know-how will make the experience educational.

Habitual users of previous years' power point presentations should take note. Such usage is becoming the bane of learning doctors' lives as a regular experience during 'formal educational' sessions. Those old and tired presentations that were never 'educational' when first produced, but merely 'informative', are recognized by learners as the stop-gaps they are, and they are labelled by outspoken learners as distinctly unprofessional.

2. Education is a 'practice' because its educational ends and virtues can *only* be realized through, and exist in, *action*, and they are themselves being continuously developed.

Commentary

Thus learners are nurtured and cultivated by educators, not treated as artifacts that can be 'made', or 'turned into the ideal end product'. You cannot 'make' a thinking surgeon or a wise doctor, you can only seek to cultivate one. And in so doing, you cannot precisely specify exactly the ends of such cultivation. (One cannot specify in April, the precise character, growth and position of the roses that will spring in July from the bush one is then pruning. One can work towards shaping the bush, and one can hope for given colour, growth, and abundant flowering on the side that faces the house — but one cannot say more.)

3. This is why experienced educators get angry when they are badgered to specify 'learning outcomes' that nail down every last detail of what the learner 'will be able to do' at the end of the programme even before it begins.

Commentary

Such learning outcomes often lead to predictability and boredom for learner and reduce the teacher's room for creativity. That way of thinking springs from a quite different view of preparing practitioners, which is based upon the values of training rather than education, and which rejects the notion that the 'growth metaphor' is a suitable analogy for an activity which is seen as mainly about being 'drilled in skills', so as to be 'safe' practitioners. But, in fact, such drilling (which 'saves practitioners from thinking') may result in more danger to patients in complex individual cases where careful thought and complex decisions are needed, and where doctors actually need to use their judgement.

4. As Carr, W. shows, to engage in an educational practice involves *more than* 'knowing how to do educational things' (having the 'skills' of teaching).

Commentary

Indeed, an educational method (like instructing doctors in a given skill) can be skilfully performed but it will not be an educational practice at all, if (for example), it has been used to impose a process upon learners who have been required to ignore their personal perspectives including their own values, attitudes and feelings, suspend their thinking, shut down their critical faculties, abandon their moral awareness, and merely parrot a performance. This would not conform to ethical educational principles of procedure concerned with cultivating the *understanding* which enables learners to explore and come to own a view about why, how, where and when to use that skill, which in turn commits them to develop or change their practice. Indeed, it would be training, not education.

Summary

From this we can see that teachers as educators in the moral mode of practice recognize the significance of developing the whole person, their understanding, their knowledge, their skills, abilities, competencies and capacities. They also recognize that deeper understanding will normally lead to commitment to the natural improvement of practice. The puzzle for the educator *then*, is how best to develop in learners the kind of understanding that is chosen for and with the learner. Two key processes in this are: to engage learners in critical thinking and to support them in making their own meaning from their experiences. Later chapters look at this in detail.

To ask what learners and teachers *generally* need to do, in order to engage learners in developing their understanding, is to ask: what principles of procedure should guide teaching activities? However, to argue for the significance of educational principles is not the same as wanting to turn them into a set of codified rules to be followed slavishly. Educational principles should guide practice in general but not shape and control it in the specific case. In the light of this the teacher needs to make wise judgements in choosing particular activities, of teaching, learning and assessment, especially tailored to the individual learner's needs (as construed and agreed by both teacher and learner). This will then lead to sound educational action. The following chapter looks at this in more detail.

Further reading

General Medical Council (2006) *Good Medical Practice*. London: GMC.

Carr, D. (2007) Character in Teaching, *British Journal of Educational Studies*. **55** (4): 369-389.

Carr, W. (1995) What is an Educational Practice? in *For Education: Towards Critical Educational Enquiry*. Buckingham: Open University Press, (chapter four).

Chapter Six

Seeing learners anew: recognizing our moral responsibilities to them

> What matters to me most [about the learners I work with] is what is at the core of their being, what my learners need to know [understand, be able to do and be] in order to become a good moral, virtuous doctor. I need to remember though that I also have a duty of care to them to ensure that all curriculum topics are covered so that they are able to complete training and pass their exit examination.
>
> Extract from the personal philosophy, written at the completion of the PG Cert by another of the consultants whose first observation was referred to in chapter one above.

Introduction
A new role for learners in postgraduate medical and surgical practice
Some important characteristics of postgraduate doctors as learners
Developing the learning doctor as a whole person
Further reading

Introduction

The comments in the box above reveal a serious paradox. The consultant sees the need to start from *where* the learner is, and *who* the learner is, and to work to facilitate their development as a person, a learner and a good clinician. Further, the learner should be a key agent in that process. The paradox is that the learner's formal curriculum, being technically oriented, does not recognize any of this as 'topics' to be taught and assessed. Thus, as a teacher who has seen the implications of the moral mode of practice, and who has a strong sense of what matters educationally to her, she also sees that this must be attended to (in terms of time and resources) either in addition to, or inside, the official curriculum to which the learner has an entitlement. In fact she goes on later to recognize the need to work to influence that formal curriculum and also to argue for more time for education. This is an example of what Palmer (1998) means by the courage needed by teachers.

Seeing the learner anew in this way, as an individual — a person who is central to her teacher's educational thinking — this consultant has established a different educational relationship from that normally found in PGME. This has created a more fruitful starting point for her teaching. The learner has been recognized as a fellow practitioner and a *person*, who has a range of needs and who also brings important contributions to the teaching. The teacher has started by studying the learner and clearly continues to do so, in order to attend to them *as a person*. The educational interaction between the two of them thus inevitably has a different dynamic from that found in much traditional PGME, where it is routinely assumed that there is no time to engage with learners in this way. In fact, as chapter ten will show, where there is improved interaction between learner and teacher as a result of establishing a sound relationship between them, their educational time can be spent more profitably.

This chapter explores a different way of seeing, understanding and inter-relating with postgraduate learners and points up the central significance for education of the teacher studying their individual learner(s), which is an activity that it sees as even more important than studying general *learning theories*. This is because no individual learner is well described by generalized theory and there is no one single overarching 'theory of learning' that encapsulates what teachers need to understand about their learners. Rather, there is only a huge range of, often contradictory, theories and ideas.

Thus, there is no substitute for meeting and getting to know each new learner as a person, as early as possible and without prior disposition to see them in any particular way beyond recognizing the teacher's responsibility to help them to achieve *their* best possible educational ends. This moral demand is exactly parallel to the doctor's responsibility to relate to each patient, irrespective of what that patient brings.

The first main section of this chapter therefore begins by exploring the new role for learners in PGME that needs to be recognized if their education is to be developed within the moral mode of practice. The second section summarizes some important characteristics of postgraduate doctors as learners. The final section then considers the importance of developing the learning doctor as a whole person and argues that, since personality and character are key elements in being a doctor, PGME teachers should seek to attend educationally to the person their learner brings to both medical practice and to their own education.

The following chapter then provides an overview of those theoretical domains that a teacher might draw upon to help them think about their learner, learning and education more generally, but which are no substitute for understanding (as far as possible) the person the teacher is working with as a learner and a doctor.

A new role for learners in postgraduate medical and surgical practice

In the purely technical mode of practice, the learner is quite simply the *object* of the teacher's work! That is, teachers in the technical mode see learners as people whose behaviour is to be shaped according to the protocols they are to be trained in, or whose knowledge can be added to through what Freire (1970) has called 'the banking concept' of education. Thus, in the technical mode of educational practice learners feature less in the teacher's thinking and in their preparation than does the protocol to be taught or the knowledge to be handed on. It is not that the teacher in this mode does not care at all for the learner. Indeed, the teacher may well believe that it is in the learner's best interests to be treated in this way and provided thus with these new skills or knowledge. It is simply that often more thought is given during the teacher's preparation — to *what the teacher will do* — than to whom the learner is as a person, (what they know, how they think, and what their personal qualities and character are). Thus for the teacher in the technical mode, the 'educational' aims are focused on what that teacher will *do to* the learner.

In this technical mode, learners almost become a *tabula rasa* on which the technically-oriented teacher expects to write. Worryingly, many consultants and senior clinicians who teach their learners knowledge and skills in the clinical setting, still broadly (if unconsciously) adopt this approach. This process, sometimes referred to as 'the transmission of knowledge', brings with it, insidiously, an attitude to learners that places them in a passive and unthinking role, and takes little account of them as people. Freire shows clearly in his work (1970 and 1998/2001) that a 'traditional transmission pedagogy' (the banking approach of imparting knowledge into the learner's storage system) can be a form of oppression, in which learners 'bank' knowledge that is alien to (incompatible with) their normal ways of thinking and understanding, because they have not made meaning out of it for themselves. They thus become 'depositories' (patiently receiving, memorizing and repeating as well as filing and storing the *teacher's* knowledge and skills), while the teacher is a 'depositor' (issuing communiqués, information and instructions and demonstrating how to do things), (see Friere 1970: 53). Freire (who was writing in a highly political context) argues that in learners this can lead to alienation and a sense of slavery. However, this is not to suggest that the teacher should never be involved in 'transmission'. For example, interacting with the learner immediately after offering them some information, can enable them to rephrase it so as to be personally more meaningful, while the teacher can listen and check that this transformation has not distorted the original meaning. Further, as Carr, D. (2003) shows, the teacher can also be a 'transmitter of moral values' (by modelling and inviting consideration of that model), and in that sense, the teacher cannot help influencing learners by their own conduct, but the intention is not to deposit knowledge but to offer examples from the teacher's own practice for consideration and critique.

By contrast, in the moral mode of practice, learners have a new role. Each one is quite simply the centre of their teacher's focus and the main subject of the teacher's study. Indeed, no educationally worthwhile aims can be formulated without looking carefully at every aspect of what the learner brings as a person to the educational interaction. Learners then become for the teacher an interest in *themselves*, a person with whom the teacher can interact collaboratively by means of a professional conversation, such that (normally) both become teachers and learners, and both benefit from greater enjoyment of the process (although learners in difficulty may sometimes need some additional approaches).

By 'professional conversation' here is meant a discussion between colleagues, (both of whom acknowledge that they are always both a teacher and a learner) that analyzes, interprets and reflects on an aspect of practice that the more junior doctor has experienced, carried out, or observed. This is not a one-way process, in which the senior teacher gives the learner feedback or a critical commentary, neither is it an interrogation by teacher of learner, as in some debriefing processes. These are activities more suitable to the technical mode of teaching. Rather, the professional conversation seeks to develop a critical appreciation of what happened and what is to be learnt from it. Here the senior doctor picks out salient points of the event and leads the learner to formulate an appreciation of what happened by examining that event from a number of perspectives. Thus, the professional conversation in which the learner works with the teacher in a nurturing environment is a cornerstone of education in the moral mode of practice, and teachers who revert to 'feedback' instead will quickly find the learner becoming defensive and less open to learning.

Using a professional conversation to formulate an appreciation of a clinical (or even an educational) event, involves collaborative analysis and interpretation in which both parties seek to consider the activity from many points of view, balancing pros and cons, seeking to set it in a context that helps to make sense of it, seeing in it meanings beyond the surface and seeing it as representative of something beyond itself. The result of this process is sometimes called 'a critical appreciation', (see Fish 1998). It can either lead the 'appreciator' more deeply into the event, or away from the activity under review towards larger matters. As such it can be a useful starting point for a teaching session with a learner in or near the clinical setting.

In the moral mode of educational practice, the teacher works *with* (not on) the learner, and in doing so meets that learner *as a whole person*. Here, learners are not buckets to be filled nor are they banks into which to deposit the teacher's wisdom, or even actors to be offered critique or feedback on what they did. Instead they are interlocutors who, *with their teacher's help*, need to make their own meaning out of new knowledge gained or an event experienced and recorded. Indeed, they are far more persuaded by exploring for themselves the knowledge on offer or the actual evidence from an observer of the event they have been engaged in, so that they come to their own recognition of what occurred. Here they will find both their achievements and their shortcomings easier to accept than ever they will by just being told about them in a 'take it or leave it' approach that can seem confrontational even when it is not intended to be so.

This is a serious change of role for both teacher and learner. It springs from an understanding that a teacher in the moral mode of practice *cultivates* learners and develops their sensitivities to people and events, rather than acting as a transmitter of information that a poor or difficult learner may then treat as mere adverse opinion. This liberates them both, so that they simultaneously become teachers and learners. To this end, teachers can adopt a range of approaches. For example, they can become the relatively humble collector of a range of data about what happens or has happened, rather than a judgemental observer, thus providing the irrefutable evidence that will enable the learner to confront for themselves the quality of their own work. By such means also, a teacher can model desirable conduct or approaches to problem solving that should enable the learner to think ideas through for themselves, and come to understand them in their own terms and language. This means that the teacher develops learners' 'power to perceive critically the way they exist in the world ... in which they find themselves', (Freire 1970: 64).

The important demand made by MMC that postgraduate doctors should become more active and pro-active as learners in the clinical setting (with its concomitant requirements of their teachers), should have made the transition from the technical to the moral mode of practice easier and more consonant with national curriculum requirements. Sadly however, such educational understanding was entirely missing from MMC and much of this way of seeing learners is even today given only lip service within many curricula, whilst not being supported by the way that the rest of the curricula are written. Thus, nowhere is there serious information for teachers about how to achieve this, and the natural processes for doing so that existed within good firms have now been lost sight of. But at least MMC's original demand leaves us with opportunities for a fuller move to the moral mode of practice in which teachers recognize their responsibility to develop the learning doctor as a whole person.

Some important characteristics of postgraduate doctors as learners

This section will offer some general principles about working with postgraduate doctors as learners in the clinical setting, within the moral mode of practice. These principles have been developed out of reflection on numerous individual experiences that have been shared with me (both in practice and as written examples) by consultants and other senior teachers who have begun to work within this mode.

Most importantly these senior doctors have learnt that attending to learners *as people in whose education they are seriously interested*, has dramatically altered for the better their teaching/learning interactions and daily working relationships. They have been particularly voluble about what a difference this makes. An example that is not untypical is to be found at the front of this chapter. It is the result of the teacher getting to know learners by meeting them as people and understanding their abilities, aspirations, values, beliefs, foibles, strengths and weaknesses and using this understanding to mediate and supplement their required curriculum. (See also Thomé 2012 and Bullock, Hardyman and Phillips 2012.)

Learners' wants and needs

Linked to this is the issue about attending to what the learner wants, and how far it is right and reasonable to divert from a planned agenda either in what is prepared by the teacher or even during a teaching session, in order to attend to learners' wants. This of course is partly a matter of judgement within each context, but it should also be influenced by the teacher's understanding of what is needed. Wilson (1971) has offered some important points that distinguish between a learner's wants and their needs. He has also demonstrated that using a learner's interests as a motivating vehicle can be beneficial. Of course this is by no means always possible, though a teacher can, with some ingenuity and creativity, sometimes shape that which they need to attend to, in ways that genuinely also meet the learner's interests.

In respect of the learner's 'wants', Wilson points out that it may well not be in the learner's best educational *interest* or in anyone else's, to pursue these. Indeed, a doctor's wants may not be in the patients' best interests either, and certainly may not be educationally worthwhile. Only the teacher is really experienced and educationally knowledgeable enough to know how appropriate or otherwise it is to pursue what the learner says they want. This is why it is better to reply to learner's questions about 'wants', with comments about their 'educational needs', and to tease apart the differences, since both teacher and learner should be able to agree on the educational needs, and they can be appropriately grounded in the context in which the learner is being taught (that is, the needs of practice, the requirements of the curriculum and what is in the best interests of patients).

The learner challenged

This will involve challenging the learner (in a nurturing environment)! In this case, the challenge is about not giving in to requests for teaching that are in some way inappropriate. This should be done unhesitatingly and with the appropriate authority and gravitas combined with a willingness to explain why the request is denied. A different form of challenge, and a more important one, is about taking the learner beyond their comfort zone intellectually in order to develop them further. I have been startled in many professional conversations with clinicians to be told that they have been discouraged from challenging or stretching learners because of their fear of being reported for bullying (which is a category that still remains on the GMC's annual evaluation questionnaire and is defined purely in the light of whether the learner 'feels' bullied, irrespective of the teacher's intention). By contrast, it is an educational principle that teaching which does not challenge will not provide the learner with intellectual stimulus, and is unlikely to be educationally worthwhile. Teachers of postgraduate doctors should be prepared to challenge learners intellectually, whilst nurturing them personally. Intellectual challenge within a positive teacher/learner relationship and in a nurturing context, is a necessary part of education, and learners rarely fail to respond to it.

Learners will respond to demands

In my experience, postgraduate doctors 'in training' are proving quick to catch on to the additional educational benefits they gain from teachers who work in the moral mode of practice. They are also quick to recognize that whilst this demands more from them, it makes learning more enjoyable and worthwhile. (See also Thomé 2012 and Bullock, Hardyman and Phillips 2012.) Thus, it should be noted, that postgraduate doctors (who under EWTD now have fewer hours in their working week than ever before) are not so overworked that they cannot engage in preparation for a teaching session or in some follow-up activities that involve them in serious writing and reading. Of course learners are more willing to write and read if the teacher routinely expects it, is equally committed to preparation and follow up, and is sure to respond further to such follow-up by their learner. Then, they will find learners more willing to write than they might expect, more willing to prepare than they might assume and more willing to read than they would have surmised. Learners asked to do these things (and who see the reason) will produce what is expected and also will quickly realize how much more they get out of the teacher's time and attention as a result. They also recognize quickly and respond enthusiastically to resources that have been created for them, that are designed to get them thinking. And this too is a way of motivating learners to do more, because the teacher has done more. (See chapter nine below.)

Particularly, I would argue, the learning doctor will respond with improved commitment when attended to by their teacher *as a whole person*. Indeed, it could be said that the PGME teacher's responsibilities are to be found centrally in working with the doctor from this basis. In the past, doctors, who treated the patient's disease but not the patient, applied the same approach to their learners. They attended to their technical needs but not to the learning doctor as a human being. In my experience as both a patient and a medical educator however, just as patients flourish more if they can meet their doctor 'whole person to whole person' (see Fish and de Cossart 2007, chapter nine), so too learning doctors respond with enthusiasm to those who are willing to support and help them as individuals while they struggle (otherwise invisibly) with meeting the demands on them as people who engage in seriously difficult professional practice. And both parties gain greater benefits as a result.

Developing the learning doctor as a whole person

Clearly then, working with 'the whole person the doctor is' can be seen to constitute an important role for the PGME teacher who certainly needs to *cultivate* learners and their sensitivities to people and events and to support them in establishing who they are, as a doctor, and a professional, and who they wish to become. Further, this is the case both for those who have recently become a practising doctor and those who are becoming more senior. Knowing who we are is an indispensible platform from which to interact with and serve vulnerable patients, to utilize wisely our skills and judgement, to respond to colleagues and managers and even to shape a career path. Finding out who we are, once we become a practising professional, what we stand for, what our aspirations really are and how these fit what we have to offer, is central to being able to engage in good practice. Coming to know oneself in this context is best done by serious and focused reflection on specific instances from our own practice, aimed at analyzing and interpreting these as fully as possible, and guided and responded to by a wise teacher (see Fish and de Cossart 2007). To an extent this can be done as part of more traditional PGME activities like case exploration — once both teacher and learner recognize that there are always two parties to a patient case (the second being the learning doctor), and that that doctor needs as much educational attention and help in exploring their own issues as the patient (normally) needs therapeutic intervention!

Thus, in working with a particular learner we need to meet them as a person and a doctor, and recognize what they bring to their learning. Here the learning agreement is the important start, and how that meeting goes will influence considerably the on-going educational relationship. Treated as a cold and speedy technical exercise, that first meeting to set the learning agreement can effectively, if inadvertently, close off the first and best opportunity for establishing a basis for the kind of relationship where both parties meet person to person, in order to engage together in the development of the whole doctor. Further, whilst such an agreement offers a start from which to attempt new achievements, it should be kept under frequent review and modifications should routinely be made in the light of what the learner actually brings, what their motivations actually are, and what they can actually do and might realistically seek to achieve. Also, attention to the formal curriculum alone does not really go far enough for those working in the moral mode of practice where the responsibility of both teacher and learner is to work on the learner's development as a whole person. In old PGME this was summed up in the idea of assessing the learner's professionalism (a term rather poorly defined in most of the documentation related to MMC), and their communication skills. As the rest of this section shows, it means far more.

Within the moral mode of practice then, where education is the intention, the purpose of PGME at any and all levels is to engage with the professional in order to nurture their human flourishing. Although this can be interpreted variously, it is meant here to indicate that PGME should centre on enabling the learner as a whole person to be the best they can be as a virtuous person and doctor. This in turn is about how they really are with patients, colleagues, managers and juniors, (not just how, on the surface, they interact with them). This relates crucially to their personality and their character, within which lie their values and beliefs, their ethical views and their moral compass. And of course, all these qualities are also crucial components of the person their teacher is, which is why 'being a teacher' makes such serious demands.

Given that the whole person (including appropriate qualities of personality, character and disposition) is what the learning doctor needs to bring to their practice, but that 'little of this is reducible to academic knowledge or technical skill' (Carr, D. 2007: 370) and given that this learner is already an adult and a practising doctor, the following questions needs to be asked. What qualities are actually constitutive of a good medical practitioner; which of these might and should the educator help to develop in the postgraduate doctor; and what kinds of development are possible in principle? Rather shockingly, even a brief survey of Good Medical Practice will indicate how startlingly lacking it is in reference to the full range of personal qualities now described below.

What qualities are actually constitutive of good medical practice?

As Carr demonstrates, teaching is 'more professionally commendable when ... carried out by those who are trustworthy, respectful of others, fair, patient, loyal, principled, discrete, responsible, conscientious, good humoured, witty, optimistic, self-restrained, persistent or lively' (Carr, D. 2007:370). He also invokes Aristotle's virtue of the mean, making the point that virtues do not lie in extremes. This is clearly true in medicine where other qualities more specific to medical practice might be added, and might be expressed in terms of moderation or temperance. Such virtues might include: exercising carefully-tempered imagination in respect of patients' perspectives; confronting and learning to cope in a balanced way with our own emotional reactions to the agonies of patients; recognizing the fragility of the human condition whilst maintaining optimism; keeping a balanced view about personal success in some areas of practice and lesser success in others; knowing when to stop; being brave about some things and fearful of others; and having respect for everyone and commitment — to patients particularly — beyond the call of duty, but also being able to balance empathy and compassion in respect of one individual with the need to preserve self for the service of others. Such a list, of course, though inevitably incomplete, might in itself be a resource for developing the ideas, self-awareness and educational agenda of young doctors.

Carr makes the point in respect of his own list (and which is also true of the medical one) that it is not totally clear which of these are qualities of character or of personality and that some overlap into both. He further suggests that 'it seems more natural to apply the language of praise and blame to qualities of character more than personality....' and adds 'whereas the qualities commonly associated with character have the moral stamp of virtues, those associated with personality have more the aesthetic flavour of personal predilection or taste' (Carr, D. 2007: 370). This suggests that whilst character might be a focus of appropriate development, personality would be less amenable to change.

Clearly there is no perfect single combination of those personal qualities that conduce to best practice, but in each of us who is successful in our professional work there are compensating qualities — which have been adopted 'precisely, by cultivating the more obviously moral qualities of character' (Carr, D. 2007: 371) — that balance our deficits, enough at least to enable us to provide a satisfactory service. Thus, he argues, 'any professional interest in character must be an interest in the cultivation of *morally good* character' (Carr, D. 2007: 372). Aristotle, he argues is '... emphatic that full acquisition of the moral virtues of courage, temperance and justice requires the principled reflection of practical wisdom' (Carr, D. 2007: 373).

Broadly then, the way we conduct ourselves in the world of our professional practice (be it in education or medicine) is arguably influenced not only by the depth of our knowledge and the excellence of our skills but also by our personal qualities. These are seated in our character, personality and dispositions, and are complemented by our intellectual abilities in interpreting the demands of the context and harnessing awareness, understanding and judgement to make an appropriate and sensitive response to the needs of learners or patients. As Carr points out:

> Aristotle's ethics is primarily an ethics of character more than of action guidance, the main role of moral reason is not the production of right actions (despite the clear moral importance of this) but the formation or cultivation of virtuous character: for Aristotle, good conduct is whatever the person of virtuous character would do.... It is clear that the virtues are not for the virtuous merely conducive to the flourishing life but *constitutive* of it.
>
> *(Carr, D. 2007: 378-9)*

This is in essence about being virtuous for its own sake and since this seems to encapsulate the kind of person in whose hands the care of vulnerable patients should be placed, it seems reasonable that the cultivation of such a *phronimon* or wise person, should be part of PGME.

Which of these can and should the educator help to develop in the postgraduate doctor?

As Carr suggests, aspects of personality are unlikely to benefit from educational development, but qualities of character are — particularly the qualities of character related to moral virtue, because they are 'not a once and for all or fixed final matter.' He adds:

> If, as Aristotle (1925: 28) points out, 'the virtues do not arise in us by nature though we are fitted by nature to receive them', it would seem to be of some general and professional importance to appreciate how we might assist the cultivation of good character.
>
> *(Carr, D. 2007: 383)*

He further argues that what is needed for the cultivation of character is 'serious reflection upon the moral purposes of human life — and upon the place of moral dispositions in achieving such purposes....' and this is possible 'only through the exercise of *phronesis*'. Since acquiring wisdom requires life-long learning, he then makes the case that such cultivation of wisdom through *phronesis* should continue beyond schooling into higher education and professional education. He emphasizes that such wisdom is absolutely distinct from, and is not acquired by, simply applying the 'right' scientific knowledge or research to a practical problem, in other words that it is not aimed at engaging in theoretical or technical enquiry, but that 'effective professional deliberation in teaching is a matter of the complex interplay of theoretical, moral and technical reflection (Carr, D. 2007: 284; and 2000: 84-5). It seems reasonable to claim beyond this, that these ideas are equally important in the cultivation of the wise doctor (see Fish and de Cossart 2007 and de Cossart and Fish 2005: 54-6).

What kinds of development are possible in principle?

David Carr argues in respect of schooling that, 'good teachers should want to cultivate a range of values and virtues that are conducive to positive and productive relations with pupils'. Indeed, he makes the point that:

> any such case for the cultivation of qualities of virtuous character as a key component of professional development is especially compelling with regard to teaching (and/or perhaps some other occupations such as ministry).
>
> *(Carr, D. 2007: 382)*

Arguably this is doubly the case for PGME, since the medical teacher will wish to establish such good relationships with the learning doctor they are responsible for, not only in order to enhance that learner's education but also in turn to develop in that learner the ability to establish good relationships with patients, colleagues and managers. (All three groups are necessary here, in order to avoid the not unfamiliar corridor complaint about a given doctor whose colleagues do not respect him but whose managers 'think he is terrific', or vice-versa!)

In principle then, the cultivation of key virtues for medical practice can often be attended to as part of other teaching — like engaging in Case Based Discussion (CBD) or Direct Observation of Procedures (DOPs) discussions — if the teacher (and learner) look for the opportunities. Some of the ways of engaging with this are gradually being more emphasized as PGME curricula develop further. Indeed, the iceberg of professional practice, as advocated in Fish and de Cossart 2007, chapter four, as prompting learners to explore the person they brought to a case or procedure under discussion, is now gaining a main place in the Foundation Curriculum. Thus medical educators do already attend to some of this, but perhaps without being totally conscious of what it is they are doing. That is why this book is about *re-focusing* rather than changing, PGME.

Two further foci in the education of the whole doctor relate to moral sensibility and sensitivity to words. These are the domain of The Arts and particularly, but not exclusively, Literature. As Carr pointed out, emotional education and development will entail changes in attitudes and values (Carr, D. 2005b: 144) for which creative and imaginative literature is the richest potential source of human normative enquiry and moral inspiration (*ibid*: 146). See also Fish 1998.

Sensitizing learning doctors to the imaginative response to 'the other' is very much about cultivating moral virtue via the arts – and through doctors' stories (see Hunter 1991, and the work of Greenhalgh; Frank; Heath; etc). Carr, W. 2005b: 148-9 talks about 'the power of art and literature, [particularly poetry], to deepen and extend our understanding of ourselves, the world and our relations with others...'. He identifies two key respects in which art and literature may help to assist the cultivation of feelings and emotions: in 'exploring the consequences for well-being and flourishing of character'; and 'choice as precisely grounded in the passions and desires of human agents'. As he argues, art is about the complexity of the human condition, about intention, and motive, and how 'bad can follow from character flaws'. In short, it is about manners and morals (Lionel Trilling, 1950, on the nineteenth century novel).

For Aristotle's views about the value of the arts – and particularly poetry — for developing moral wisdom, see his *Poetics*, where he maintains that poetry offers greater insight into the human experience than philosophy or history, because it portrays universal human predicaments and associated emotions through stories and themes. Such art (stories in words, pictures, drama, dance, poetry, music) offers us striking and memorable images that place us as readers vividly in a situation that touches us individually, and calls for our full human response. Such exercising of the imagination extends our wisdom and its role in professional practice. As Carr says:

> Such broader wisdom and understanding is also often evident in deeper and more sensitive appreciation of the complexities of human association, greater awareness of and sympathy for

the differing circumstances of others, and correspondingly enhanced interpersonal capacities.

(Carr, D. 2007: 386)

In the light of this, the current vogue of sending young doctors on a communication skills course to equip them better to break bad news seems utterly crass. Hence, as Carr usefully concludes:

> Hence, although it would also be mistaken to hold that their [the Arts'] value is entirely exhausted by their moral import, the central role of literature and the arts in any process of moral formation — properly conceived as an education of the heart as well as the head – would seem hard to deny.
>
> *(Carr, D. 2005b: 150)*

For an excellent volume on professional character development and medical education, see Kenny and Shelton (eds) (2006). This contains chapters on character formation (Veatch; Pellegrino; and Mann).

Another important and allied quality in young doctors is sensitivity to the nuance of words, and the power of different discourses to make us see in particular ways and to accept (or make) distorted arguments. This can be achieved by looking at the language used (talking, reading and writing) and at the discourse in the clinical setting, in different departments and healthcare professions, and also in the hospital at large. The area within educational literature known as 'Language in Education' contains (as we shall see) a range of useful principles for working with teachers in the four modes of language to develop their sensitivity to words and to the importance of being aware of a variety of discourses.

This chapter then has tackled some issues about educating the learner by drawing on practical experience about learners in PGME. However, there is much more to be said about them since, being at the centre of all education, they can be seen behind most, if not all, the chapters in this book. More practical details about working with learning doctors are to be found in chapter ten. Perspectives from educational theories that offer some light on learning and by implication, teaching, can be found in chapter seven, which now follows.

Further reading

* Carr, D. (2000) *Professionalism and Ethics in Teaching*. London: Routledge (chapter five).

Carr, D. (2005b) On the contribution of literature and the arts to the educational cultivation of moral virtue, feeling and emotion, *Journal of Moral education*, Vol. **34** (2): 137-151.

Fish, D. (1998) *Appreciating Practice in the Caring Professions*. London: Heinemann

Fish, D. and de Cossart L. (2007) *Developing the Wise Doctor*. London: RSM Press (chapter four).

Chapter Seven

Seeing educational theory anew: exploring its nature and purpose

As Carr, D. points out, educational theory is not the same *kind* of theory as medical theory. He also says:

> although it is hardly reasonable to suppose that one might practice medicine in the absence of considerable knowledge of such sciences as anatomy or physiology, it is less easy to see what sorts of studies might provide precisely analogous theoretical input to effective educational practice.

(Carr, D. 2003:53)

He argues rather for principled reflection on and deep deliberation about our own practice and in what sense it is educationally worthwhile, rather than being in thrall to a particular aspect of one theoretical discipline that happens to interest us, and seeking uncritically to inject the influence of that into our work.

He also argues that: 'there could hardly be any other professional field in which there is as wide disagreement about the purpose, value and utility of theory in professional training as there is in the field of teacher education and training'.

(Carr, D. 2000:65)

Introduction
An exploration and refutation of some false assumptions
Considering the nature and purpose of educational theory
The main constituents of formal educational theory
Theories that underpin this book's view of learning and teaching
The centrality of language to learning
The vital importance of clinical reflection as central to learning in PGME
Further reading

Introduction

This chapter sets out to explore the complex nature of educational theory, consider how it relates to the practices of teaching and education and establish how, for what purpose, and in what way, a teacher might actually use it. Firstly, however a ground-clearing exercise is necessary in order that doctors seeking to become enhanced teachers do not falsely equate 'quality in teaching' with the need to acquire 'the whole' of educational theory in order to apply it to practice. The aim here is rather that readers come to recognize the many different 'ways of knowing', (kinds of evidence, view of 'truth', and structuring concepts) that lie within the range of academic disciplines that loosely make up educational theory, and understand that such theory, being generalized, will not fit individual practice. To this end, this chapter is structured in six sections. Following the ground clearing, section two explores the nature of educational theory and section three offers an overview of theory's main components. The main theoretical influences on this book as a whole are then reviewed, and the chapter ends by highlighting two important components of theory: language in learning and clinical reflection.

An exploration and refutation of some false assumptions

The comments in the box at the front of this chapter contain a major warning to doctors who — in wishing to learn to improve their teaching or to think better about education — inevitably come with expectations endemic to the practice of medicine, that they will need to learn 'the' education theory as a basis for their practical teaching. This assumption contains at least three misconceptions, each underpinned by the idea that education as a *theoretical* discipline provides us with a particular 'way of knowing' (see Phenix 1964) that will directly inform educational practice in the same way that theoretical knowledge of human systems directly informs medical practice. Thus, whilst the practice of education shares many parallels with the practice of medicine, its theoretical basis differs in *kind and character* from the nature of medical knowledge, and it plays a different role in relation to practice.

Firstly, it is a misconception or perhaps a false assumption that there actually is one integrated and commonly accepted, official and formal theoretical basis for education — A Grand Theory of Education — made up of commonly agreed subsections, all of which will inform us about what is correct teaching or tell the teacher how to teach. That is simply wrong! There is no singular and all-embracing Education Theory that informs and validates educational practice. Rather there are many different theoretical fields that offer the teacher a range of very different perspectives on education or on teaching, learning and assessment generally. But in no case does any of these offer the practising teacher clear and incontrovertible laws about how to proceed in their specific practice with their specific learner. They are not about 'how to teach' in the way that a surgical textbook may be about 'how to do a particular kind of operation'. Therefore none has a direct claim above the others to be learnt and applied throughout educational practice. And further, none can offer a specific and agreed standard or 'norm' in respect of 'the best way to teach'.

By contrast, while it might be said of Medical Theory that there are also many branches of it (as in anatomy, physiology, histopathology), these empirical sciences play a more clear-cut role in medical practice because they provide incontrovertible knowledge of 'the normal' in bodily structure and disease-free life. Thus, medical undergraduates learn empirical knowledge from several disciplines as a resource in order to understand the normal and to know when something is not normal in order to work back to the normal. That is, would-be doctors learn medical theory in order to apply it in practice. Further, this theory provides them with an agreed 'norm' that is understood across all medical practice.

Secondly, there is a misconception about what theoretical basis a teacher can claim in support of their practice, whereas there is no dispute about the theoretical bases of a doctor's practice. Thus, medical practice makes much of the idea that it is based on 'objective knowledge', drawing on science, and being research- or evidence-based, but it is out of ignorance of the nature of educational theory and practice that PGME asks it to do the same for teaching. In fact, of course, when pressed, doctors do recognize that medicine as a practice is at heart an interpretive or subjective practice because a doctor tailors general science to individual human differences, and is dependent for this on professional judgement that actually is values-based! (See, for example, Hunter 1991 and Montgomery 2006.)

Unlike medical practice therefore, educational practice cannot even begin to claim a sound scientific or research basis that teachers must conform to. It is not 'theory-based' but rather 'values-based'. Indeed, a teacher's practice is based more upon commonly agreed principles of practice (theorized from practice). This, for each specific teaching event, may be supported by theoretical underpinnings drawn from a range of theoretical perspectives, but even the choice of that is influenced by the teacher's personal values and the context in which they are working. This does not mean, as some like Carr W. seem to claim, that education is totally problematic because there is no serious consensus about best practice amongst experienced educators. But it does mean that specific educational practices are recognized 'up-front' as unable to be 'proved' by reference to grand theory. They rest rather on a form of *critical appreciation* that I have elsewhere referred to, quoting Armstrong 1996), as 'Venetian Justification', and 'Intersubjective Validity' (see Fish 1998).

These terms are Armstrong's way of explaining connoisseurship in the Arts. But they are also useful in providing evidence for the quality of practical education. Here, too, there is no single prime basis to support and *justify* the quality of our educational practice, as in a particular teaching event (though we may gain some empirical evidence through assessment processes about what the learners have gained as a result). Rather the evidence for recognizing success and probity in educational practice comes through lots of small points drawn from the networks and practices of educational theory and practice traditions, 'none of which is decisive on its own, but cumulatively they approach justification', Armstrong (1996): 151, quoted in Fish (1998): 253. Armstrong calls this Venetian Justification because Venice is not built on solid ground but is supported by millions of wooden piles or piers driven into the lagoon and, although not one of these alone supports the buildings, 'the multiplicity of little supports allows us to approach security'. Thus the justification of good educational practice is supported by many piers. Further, Armstrong argues, where work sustains the judgement that it is of high merit on similar grounds across a wider range of judges, we can see that judgement as Inter-subjectively Valid even if some few disagree, (*ibid*). In time, such connoisseurship develops a more and more discriminating and refined palate, so that educators can come to a substantial consensus about a specific event, but it will still not be possible to write a general protocol to ensure quality teaching in all contexts.

Teaching is therefore an activity driven not as in medicine by 'the book that currently everyone uses', but more by critical and reflective enquiry into practice by the teacher, who, sometimes with other colleagues, draws upon and *thinks with* a range of theoretical perspectives, and for whom there neither is, nor ever will be, 'the' textbook. Thus, although at the point of engaging in practice, doctors and teachers are very similar because both rely in the end on sound professional judgement about what is best for the individual (patient or learner), the nature of the theoretical basis that each can cite and rely on to support and validate their professional actions differs considerably in kind.

Thirdly given the above points, it would also be an especially dangerous misconception to believe that learning to be a teacher (or better, an educator) is about learning education theory in order to *apply it to* practice. Rather, the relationship to practice of each of the very different academic educational fields means that, at best, the teacher might draw some general enlightenment about an aspect of their work, from a variety of sources, but with no guarantee that these generalizations have special relevance to the individual learner or teacher, or the specific context in which they are working. What the teacher needs then, is an overall understanding of the nature of a whole range of theoretical disciplines, and a grasp of what purposes each may serve in thinking about education.

Thus, it is clearly not possible to be a good teacher by reading and applying a few theoretical texts. Indeed, as Carr argues so eloquently:

> although it is difficult to see how anyone might be a successful surgeon or a general medical practitioner in the absence of some knowledge of anatomy or physiology, it seems perfectly conceivable that someone might be an effective teacher in the absence of any formal knowledge of psychology or sociology whatsoever.
>
> *(Carr, D. 2003: 54).*

He also says elsewhere: 'The point is not just that one cannot *sufficiently* account for professional expertise in terms of any ... technical application of theoretical knowledge, but ... that there would be no need for professional — medical, legal or educational — judgement if one could' (Carr, D. 2000: 48-9). Further, ... it is because there is no certain and significant public agreement about the aims and purposes of education and their contribution to human flourishing that 'there can be no straightforward technical or technicist construal of professional practice and professional deliberation', (*ibid*: 49). For an opposite view, see Gunderman (2006), particularly chapters 2, 3 and 4.

What educational theory can do, then, in relation to practice, is not to offer any sort of objective theory to support a specific event, but to enlighten the teacher's *thinking* (through deliberation and reflection) about a specific piece of practice — before, during and after that event — or about teaching as a practice more generally. For this to be possible, a teacher must understand the nature of educational theory and practice and in what sense it is appropriate to fuel the teacher's thinking, and they should not be seduced into seeing their educational practice from only one perspective.

Considering the nature and purpose of educational theory

Smith sees educational theory as an entitlement to understanding, not as a reservoir of academic knowledge with which to equip the practising teacher but more as a wide field of which the teacher needs a sound overview. For, he says:

> it is where there is insufficient critical, analytical thinking that the dreary orthodoxies take root and the ghosts of dead theories roam unchecked. Unless teachers have sufficient understanding of the philosophies that are *pre-supposed* by what is taken as evidence, the scope of their reflectivity, and thus their capacity for change, is limited from the outset, and they are condemned to remain second-class citizens in the world of ideas.
>
> *(Smith 1992: 391)*

He also argues that some kind of theory is implicit in all practice and that, 'all practice, as practice, is seen in the light of a perspective or theory' (Smith 1992: 389). He adds that 'the root meaning of *theory* connects it with *viewing*, and with the idea of *perceiving-as*', and adds that: 'there is no *practice* in human affairs that does not come to us filtered through one set of lenses or another', (*ibid*). But the individual teacher's lenses are made up of a mixture of personal values and chosen theoretical perspectives. He usefully offers five vital purposes of academic theory, which, as adapted to PGME, are:

▷ to challenge our current implicit and explicit theories

▷ to show that things can be otherwise

▷ to develop a sense of the nature of education

▷ to create an intelligent and well-informed faculty of teachers [of, in our case, postgraduate doctors]

▷ to make education more interesting because it becomes more intellectually challenging.

(See Smith 1992: 395-97)

Teachers, Smith argues, have an entitlement to educational theory. For postgraduate medical educators, this is because they need to: be aware of the significance of educational theory and have a grasp of its complex relationship to practice; understand the landscape of educational theory, so as to place any theory they are considering within its proper context; and remember to test theory against practice as well as to consider their practice in the light of theory.

The main constituents of formal educational theory

A wide range of disciplines from a diverse set of fields each provide a specific kind of theoretical perspective on educational practice. Their structural components, ways of knowing, attitudes to truth and methods of proof are each very different. Some fields, for example, are empirical (like educational psychology, sociology of education and linguistics), some pseudo-empirical (for example, language studies, or curriculum studies), some arts-based (like the history of education, or The Arts as in Literature, which help us understand ourselves as professionals), and some are more distinctly theoretical as in Aristotle's *Theoria* (for example, philosophy). Clearly no teacher can become an expert in all these but rather needs to understand how each field works, how to navigate it, and what kind of thinking it contributes to broad themes like teaching, learning and assessment.

Empirical disciplines

Formal educational theory from the empirical disciplines of psychology and sociology, or even linguistics, can offer us empirical data that involves generalization and claims objectivity, but which, while it may shed some light on learning more generally, cannot be relied on for help in understanding real learners! The structural bases, ways of knowing, and views about data, truth and objectivity as enshrined in these disciplines will be very familiar to any doctor. Sadly, they are the basis on which almost all educational research in medicine has been designed, even though empirical data are often not useful for teachers on the ground. This is because the empirics provide generalizations and trends, but exactly how a practising teacher should draw upon them in relation to their specific practice, is problematic. By contrast, Curriculum Studies (which Carr, D. calls a pseudo science), may have more to offer the teacher and be less purely technical than he suggests. Readers should consult Carr, D. (2000) Part Two, and (2003) Part Two, for further information.

Curriculum Studies

Although major curriculum design and development has long since been superseded in our schools by the National Curriculum, this useful field still has important insights to offer doctors, particularly in postgraduate medical education, in developing a critique of the values base, defining the nature of medical practice, and designing specialty curricula.

Understanding how a curriculum for medical practice should be set out (see Fish and Coles 2005), can help educators of postgraduate doctors to understand why they find so uncomfortable the formal curriculum of which they (wrongly) see themselves as hapless and helpless agents. This will enable them to find ways of enriching their own specialty curricula such that they can offer better versions of what they have always known was important — but which their current curricula ignore. It will also provide them with further educational support for placing learners in a more central role within their education.

The work of Stenhouse (1975) is germinal here. His three models of teaching show clearly some very different, if stereotyped, ways of construing teaching. The 'product model' emphasizes the importance of the end product of teaching, which itself is about depositing knowledge into learners. The process model emphasizes the learning processes, and sees learners as active. By extension, the research model of education, sees both teacher and learner as collaborative learners in exploring issues that are based in practice. It would seem, intuitively perhaps, that the first of these models (the product model) might be of some use in teaching new knowledge; that the second (the process model) might be more appropriate for those learning a practice: and that the third (the research model) might be the most appropriate for learners who are already postgraduate practitioners and whose work needs to be transformative of current traditions rather than replicating old ideas. None of these models however can ever exist alone and in purist fashion. Rather, Stenhouse offers important ideas about what and how to teach. See below p. 149 for more details.

Practice theorized

Practice that has had its underpinning ideas exposed (known as 'theorized practice' or practice that has been theorized), involves exploring practice, so that the theory it is based on can be made to emerge from it. This may involve teachers exploring their own practice and the responses of their learners reflectively and deliberatively in the light of a range of other ways of seeing it, or it may result from teachers acting more directly as 'insider researchers', investigating their own practice through a variety of research processes. The purpose here is to determine what ideas, beliefs, values and even assumptions drive that practice and, where appropriate, to clarify the principles upon which the practice rests.

Philosophy as useful to teachers

Different again are the perspectives offered from within that part of philosophy that is about clarifying ideas and concepts and distinguishing carefully between words that seem on the surface to be similar. These are likely to be useful to aid teachers' thinking about their practice and about the nature of knowledge, see for example Grundy (1987), Habermas (1974), Popper (2002) and Quirk (2006). Of these Quirk's ideas about the role of intuition and metacognition in medical education are perhaps the most interesting. It is philosophy, too, that lies at the basis of the formulation of the arguments about the moral mode of practice, which helps to clarify the distinctions between that and the technical mode, and enables us to examine the grounds of these claims and the basis of the moral authority of the teacher (see Carr, D. 2003, chapter five). Carr's work and the work of, for example, Hirst and Peters, also explores many associated concepts like liberalism, justice, equality, difference, freedom, authority and discipline (see Carr, D. 2003 chapters 11 – 14). Particularly helpful too, as a model, is the rigorous logic with which philosophers seek to present their arguments, and reflect on, deliberate about and critique ideas about practice. Philosophy also offers useful critical perspectives on other theoretical disciplines that influence education, like psychology and sociology, as the following sub-section shows. Philosophy, of course, in no way purports to tell people how to do something, but Passmore (1981) does open up practical ideas about fostering creativity and criticality.

Several theoretical approaches to learning

There are many different definitions of learning, stemming from very different ways of thinking about educational practice. Each carries inside it a set of beliefs and values about people and about education. *Frame 7.1 Three sample definitions of learning* offers just three different approaches to education.

Frame 7.1 Three sample definitions of learning

1. A classical behaviourist's definition

Learning is about being practised (or rehearsed) in an activity, and being rewarded for correct behaviour, until the actions learnt can be carried out on demand in the same way every time. Learning thus results from demonstration followed by practice with feedback until this leads to the permanent change in the learner's behaviour as desired by the teacher — usually in the role of an agent of some greater authority. Here, learning involves re-organization of the learner's habits, skills, tendencies, and his/her relationship with his/her environment. Little or no additional cerebral activity is required. The sign of such learning is a change in the learner's performance, which must be visible and measurable. (See for example, Pavlov, Thorndyke, Watson, Skinner, Gagné.)

2. Some philosophers' definitions

Learning is a complex activity in which we come to know ourselves and the world around us. Its achievements range from merely being aware, to what may be called understanding and being able to explain. It is both the acquisition of knowledge and the extensions of the ability to learn. It engages the learner in an on-going conversation with their heritage and culture. It is about cultivating the flourishing of a human being. (See Aristotle, Oakeshott.)

3. My definition as a medical educator

Learning is about expanding and deepening understanding. In postgraduate medicine this involves developing the whole doctor, since it is the whole doctor who should meet and care for the patient. In addition to learning to develop the appropriate and important knowledge and skills, learning in PGME should therefore also involve developing wisdom, judgement and decision-making as well as professionalism, moral awareness and sensibilities, and qualities of character that are endemic to good medical practice. This will involve liberation from narrow ways of thinking into an open-minded yet critical approach to new ideas and activities. Learning in this sense is about the learner discovering and making sense of what is important, re-thinking what is valuable, considering how this relates to their currently held values and beliefs, and whether and how it can contribute to practical ways forward. This emancipated understanding will ultimately lead to a change in the way learners conduct themselves in practice, and contribute to their personal flourishing and, as a result, to the patient's greater well-being. (See Fish and de Cossart.)

The first of the above examples fits the technical mode of practice, which is not surprising since training is the province of behavioural psychologists who value the manipulation of behaviour in animals and humans. Their view is that learning is about changing the learner's behaviour, which is initially rewarded so that the change becomes unthinkingly embedded in the learner, and proved through immediate testing.

By contrast to this behaviourist view, the second definition (a summary of the standpoint of two philosophers), is far broader and seems to value the development in the learner of a range of liberal qualities, by means of the cultivation and nurturing of their character, personal qualities, abilities, capacities, competence, beliefs, attitudes and values. This view of education regards the change of conduct and development of character as the result of changed understanding. These are rather deeper concepts, as we have seen earlier, which may not be achieved instantly or be immediately visible, since education affects both the mind and character, and reveals itself visibly, only after a period of time, in how we comport ourselves. None of this kind of learning is measurable, though it can be evidenced by demonstrating the change and development over time of the learner's thinking, and will often be clearly evident to, and appreciated by, those around them.

At first the 'medical educator's definition' (the third definition) may seem to lie at the other extreme from the behaviourists' approach, being too broad to be encompassed within, and too general to direct education in, medical practice. On closer inspection however, it encompasses more of the second than might have been expected. It is, of course, one definition — not *the* definition — offered from within the moral mode of practice, and concerned with the development of the whole doctor. Readers are invited to reflect upon these ideas and recognize that different theoretical perspectives offer deeply different views. They should then begin, as a PGME teacher, to develop their own preferred definition of learning — by studying their learners and considering their own educational practice. Having done so, they should then consider critically their own definition and identify its underlying values.

Having placed formal educational theory in its wider theoretical context of various senses of theory, it is also important to make clear the theoretical bases of this book.

Theories that underpin this book's view of learning and teaching

The main underpinning theoretical basis of this book is derived from philosophy, and particularly from Aristotelian philosophy in respect of *praxis* (see above, pp. 40-41), and the exposition and elaboration of these ideas and their implications as found in the work of Carr, D. When explored in terms of teaching and learning, arguments in Aristotle's *Ethics* lead us to see that the moral duty of the expert educator, as their own agent, is to review the possibilities for supporting the learner and choose the best for that learner. This means, as we have seen, firstly that the teacher should study the learner (the learner's needs, interests, and abilities and the context of learning). Secondly, in the light of this, the teacher should study the learner's curriculum on paper, so as to 'translate' it, or emancipate and transform it, into the best 'curriculum on the ground' for that learner. Thirdly, it means that the teacher should be aware of the range of possible theoretical perspectives on learners and learning and on teaching, such that they remain their own agent in respect of making principled choices with and for each learner as they work with them, *without becoming the agent of any one learning theory.* To ensure that their decisions are sound and continue to focus on what is best for the learner, the teacher also needs to engage in careful deliberation about and reflection on their choices as well as on the teaching and learning event and its achievements. This approach is referred to as working within a virtues-based rather than a knowledge-centred, competency-based curriculum.

Broadly there are six other main theoretical *influences* on how this book construes learning in medical practice. These are:

▶ *the behaviourist view of learning,* which this book explicitly rejects as the basis for medical education

▶ *some parts of the constructivist view of learning,* which construes the relationship between learning, language and knowledge as interactive because learners need to be 'meaning-makers' who re-make the knowledge they are offered by the teacher into their own understanding, as expressed in their own language and as relating to their own previous knowledge and experience (which this book regards as useful in balance with the following)

▶ *the socio-cultural view of learning,* which recognizes that the mind of the learner is shaped by their cultural, historical and institutional setting and that concepts and knowledge are socially acquired and socially determined (which this book respects)

▶ *the 'process' and 'research' models of curriculum design,* which inform the understanding of an approach to designing educational sessions, which encourages the development of creative new pedagogies that will transform outdated practice (which this book would wish to foster)

▶ *the 'Language in Education' approach,* which recognizes that language is the central vehicle of teaching and learning, which recognizes the importance of the learner's interaction with the teacher, and the teacher's responsibility to foster that (which this book supports, as seen in what now follows)

▶ *the literature on reflection as central to learning through experience* which for medical practitioners needs to be related to and support their clinical thinking and professional development, and which this book regards as central.

The last two will now be explored in detail as the most important in this list.

The centrality of language to learning

This section draws on ideas from Language in Education and particularly the Oracy Project of 1995 in which teachers researched with Language in Education specialists how best to enhance the interaction between teachers and learners in schools (see Norman (ed) 1995). A moment's thought will confirm that language is the central vehicle for all teaching and learning. This means that all learning is mediated through language (talking, listening, reading and writing). This is not well understood in the technical mode of practice where the teacher predominantly talks and the learner predominantly listens, where writing is rarely engaged in and reading is almost always focused on the clinical task in hand or the skill to be learned. Teachers in this mode of practice construe teaching as mainly a presentational act, in which they show learners what they know. This way of working deprives learners of their main means to explore, construct and check out what they have gained from the time they spend with their teachers.

In the moral mode of practice, however, teaching and learning are crucially seen as collaborative and exploratory. It is recognized that the learning doctor's 'meaning-making' occurs through purposeful linguistic interaction with their teachers and other colleagues. This process is commonly called the co-construction of knowledge. Through this process learners take over the teacher's understandings and resources and make them their own. They do so through purposeful discussion during which learners both create their own ways of articulating what the teacher has offered and also investigate whether this is an accurate or even an enriched version of what has been said.

The meaning-making process is referred to as 'appropriation' and involves the active transformation by the learner of the information provided by the teacher and other participants in the educational activity. Thus the learner's resulting knowledge (or understanding) is never a copy of what was initially offered, but rather a personal reconstruction. As a result it may go beyond the initial 'model' offered and learners may find new meanings and solutions to problems and even formulate new problems. These need to be shared with the teacher, and the teacher needs to listen carefully and respond to them seriously, because however much learners seem to be speaking the same language as the teacher, this does not automatically mean a shared understanding. Teachers need to remember that different life experiences, concerns and interests lie beneath a commonality of language and that these put a different interpretive gloss on the meanings of the words that have apparently been shared. Thus, participants who engage in talking together will all have to work to achieve and maintain a shared *intersubjective* understanding of the matter in hand. This takes time and patience and requires us to be able to see as the other person sees. Since this is important and also requires specialist educational knowledge and skill on the part of the teacher, the following explores this further.

The co-construction of knowledge

Mercer (1995), who was also associated with the Oracy Project, draws our attention to many of the following points. He begins by looking at where knowledge resides and who owns it. He argues that knowledge exists in the thoughts of individual people, but it is also a joint possession, and can effectively be shared (so we do not each have to re-invent the wheel). Thus we pool our mental resources to solve problems, create knowledge, and learn. He also notes that: 'One result of many heads contributing to the construction of knowledge is the vast dynamic resource we call 'culture', (Mercer (1995:2). However, as we have said, we also have to bear in mind the problem that in sharing knowledge people can also misunderstand each other. Knowledge is socially constructed. Interest in this whole area is referred to as the socio-cultural approach to thinking about learning and this sees language as a social mode of thinking.

If we see teachers as having the responsibility of helping others to construct understanding, we also recognize that talk between teacher and learner is a major means of doing this. Often teachers' talk is a means of telling learners what to do; and how to do it; when to start and stop. But actually as teachers we also need to provide experiences and resources for the learner to grapple with orally, as we, the teacher, listen. Teacher's talk then, is used to guide the co-construction of knowledge. Importantly also, we need to help learners to shape *their* representations of reality and interpretations of experience. From this teachers can learn about *them* and thus learn to help them. All learning environments thus need to provide for the re-construction of knowledge. Lecture rooms do not do this because their shape precludes detailed conversation with learners. But there is more.

Many educational uses of talking and listening

In the clinical setting we also assess learners through talking and listening (rather more than in writing, though we could ask for writing as follow-up or preparation). This ignores the great potential of learners' own writing to evidence their own achievements. We also sometimes talk of language as 'communicating', but it is also used for *thinking*... and the two really go together. Thus, conversations can be used to develop thinking — both our own and others'. Teachers can also offer language that enables learners to re-shape their thinking (and their understanding and knowing). By using language to think and learn, we also change our language. So, since it is dynamic and endlessly developing, language should not be regarded as 'a mere tool'. Teachers use language techniques to help develop a shared version of knowledge. Learners are therefore 'shaped' by the teacher's language, but also influence the teacher's language and thinking.

One of the most important uses of the learner's time and oral and written abilities is to reflect orally with, and in writing for, their teachers. A requirement to reflect on their practice is made of all postgraduate doctors and records of their reflective writing are required in learning portfolios, for appraisal purposes and in the resulting re-validation process. This is because only in-depth reflection by the doctor on particular patient cases and clinical events can reveal the quality of their professionalism, and the development and expertise of their knowledge, thinking, decision-making and professional judgements. Reflection is only just beginning to be recognized as central to sound PGME. The following section seeks to demonstrate both why this has been slow to take off and what reflection offers practising doctors.

The vital importance of clinical reflection as central to learning in PGME

In offering an introduction to reflection which has been carefully customized to doctors and their teachers, the following attends to: why reflection matters; what is involved in developing the wise doctor; what is involved in clinical reflection; and where the idea of reflection has come from. Detailed resources to help doctors reflect more deeply and purposefully will be published shortly, by Aneumi Publications in a new series entitled: Resources for doctors teaching in the clinical setting.

Why does clinical reflection matter?

Reflection is a disciplined process of investigating specific examples of one's own practice in order to make greater sense of it and to learn from it. Within the technical mode of practice serious and rigorous reflection is not well appreciated. Here, learners are not encouraged to think about and explore in their own words their personal clinical experiences. In a training context, the necessary knowledge and skills are inculcated into the learner by the trainer, and the personal aspects that colour learning are not significant. Hence the only questions asked during training in a procedure are about 'the doing', rather than what lies under that doing. A typical mantra is concerned with what the learner did well, or badly, rather than on the understanding that drives that doing. This may account for the slowness of PGME to recognize the value of reflection. It has also been seen as a 'fluffy' activity, engaged in mainly by non-medical healthcare practitioners — who do indeed mostly reflect in descriptive narrative on what they have done, rather than on the analysis and interpretation that lies beneath this.

In fact reflection is far from easy and simple. For medical educators in the moral mode of practice, reflection focuses on the detail of clinical practice, which I shall therefore refer to as *clinical reflection*. This form of reflection is central to learning in medicine. It occurs through discussion with the teacher and also in the subsequent extension of these ideas, through writing. It can occur, as Schön (1987) has taught us, both during the event ('reflection-in-action) and after the event (reflection-on-action). Boud (1985) has also pinpointed the importance of reflection *before* action (sometimes in surgery this is referred to as 'rehearsing in the mind' the surgical procedure). Clinical reflection clarifies and deepens the meaning of the clinical event or experience. Such reflection is what renders educationally worthwhile the professional conversation about practice between the teacher and learning doctor. Here, rather than merely telling a story about 'what we did' (reporting our behaviour, which is still the tendency in much healthcare practice), we should engage in properly rigorous reflection which is more 'mindful', and uncovers the drivers of personal professional practice through a three-dimensional analysis and interpretation of our conduct, considered in the light of appropriately related theory. Thus, rigorous reflection provides educational insights in a way that nothing else can and provides the key to developing the wise doctor.

What is involved in developing the wise doctor

Developing the Wise Doctor, offers resources, frameworks and language to enable doctors to reflect in this way on their practice. (See Fish and de Cossart 2007.) For such doctors, clinical reflection involves:

▷ a rigorous investigation of their own medical practice which extracts the meaning from the experience and, in making it explicit, enables it to be explored and understood

▷ focusing on their own practice and themselves as professionals and seeing themselves as learning doctors whose educational needs are as important as the needs of the patients with whom they are partners in the case

▷ seeking, in reference to specific examples of individual patient cases, events, and processes in their own practice, to uncover rigorously and to understand and articulate the relationship between their personal visions, values and beliefs, and their actual thinking, knowledge and action, and consider these in relation to the current understandings of such matters within the wider practice world

▷ exploring and providing evidence of the complexity of their practice and the quality of their expertise, which should be available (made properly anonymous) to a wider audience as well as being used for personal education.

For all this to be properly educational, of course, there needs to be a change of mindset in the medical world about blame and error, such that events that have a negative dimension can be properly aired and learnt from without fear, and those who are honest about their achievements are honoured more than those who only engage in 'impression management' about their practice.

Reflection needs to become a central process in PGME because of what it enables learners to achieve in collaboration with their teachers (who also need to become familiar with reflecting during and after their own practice).

Where has reflection come from?

Being a form of practice, the reflective process has commonly been referred to as 'reflective practice'. Key writers in this field are Dewey and Schön (1987), but contributions have also been made, for example, by Boud, in Boud, Kehoe and Walker (1995); Bolton (2010); Moon (1999); and Tripp (1993).

Reflective practice is allied to the Aristotelian view of *praxis*, which is about morally informed action, or action shaped by critical consideration of both its ends and means. Reflective practice thus involves systematic critical enquiry into one's professional work and one's relationship to it. This involves standing back from that practice (and ourselves as part of that practice) and viewing — as an observer might — and critiquing both the practice and what lies under that practice (our beliefs, assumptions, expectations, feelings, attitudes and values as they impact on our practice). Reflection, like *praxis* thrives in the moral mode of practice.

What exactly does reflection achieve?

Without reflection it would be possible to have 'the experience without the meaning' (T.S.Eliot, in *Four Quartets*). Indeed, experience alone is not the best means through which professionals learn to practice. It is the *reflection on that experience*, guided by a more experienced professional, that actually educates them. Thus, reflection on examples of their medical practice will enable any doctor to uncover rigorously, and understand and articulate the *relationship* between their visions, values and beliefs, and their thought, knowledge and action as evidenced in that practice. By 'rigorous' here is meant: being systematic, thorough and careful by using appropriately and in logical order all the perspectives available to enhance understanding. A process of Clinical Reflective Writing (CRW) has been developed by Fish and de Cossart, and the process and examples of the writing itself are currently to be found at: www. ED4MEDPRAC.co.uk.

Reflection, then, enables learners (*in respect of selected events of practice*) to:

▷ explore, make sense of, and thus understand more fully their experience, actions and events

▷ contextualize this current experience and relate it critically to other relevant theory and practice

▷ extend their current competence in clinical practice

▷ recognize new challenges to work on within clinical practice

▷ appreciate the subtleties of clinical practice

▷ connect particular practice experiences, events and activities to wider ideas and ideals of practice across their profession

▷ develop a personal vision of clinical practice

▷ provide evidence of growing insight and progress in understanding

▷ crystallize and summarize progress at the end of various stages of learning.

These perspectives will be used in Part Two to enlighten our examination of educational practice in PGME. Before that, however it is important to understand some key issues relating to the assessment of postgraduate doctors.

Further reading

* Carr, D. (2003) *Making sense of education: An introduction to the philosophy and theory of education and teaching.* London: RoutledgeFalmer. (Chapter two.)

Norman, K. (ed) (1995) *Thinking Voices: The work of the National Oracy Project.* London: Hodder & Stoughton. (Chapters 3.1 and 4.5.)

* Oakeshott, M. (1967) Learning and Teaching, in R.S. Peters (ed) *The Concept of Education.* London: Routledge and Kegan Paul.

* Schön, D. (1987) *Educating the Reflective Practitioner.* New York: Jossey Bass. (Chapters one and two.)

* Smith, R. (1992) Theory: an entitlement to understanding, *Cambridge Journal of Education,* **22** (3): 386-398.

Chapter Eight

Seeing assessment anew: re-asserting its educational role

> Thanks to 'diploma disease' [the chasing of qualifications for instrumental ends], educational systems in virtually every country are to a greater or lesser extent being deflected from their true purpose of promoting education ... into a punishing and more or less irrelevant paper chase in which few will win and many must fail.
>
> *(Broadfoot 2002: 203)*
>
> In this paper I argue that a great deal of the edifice of educational measurement is actually rooted in myth... [which is] a manifestation of the culture and power structures of our contemporary society.
>
> *(Ibid: 206).*
>
> First, educational assessment can never be scientific; and thus, second, so-called psychometric tests can never be totally objective in the way that is claimed for them.
>
> *(Ibid: 215).*
>
> In short, the myth of measurement has inhibited the positive and creative use of assessment to *promote*, rather than to *measure*, learning.
>
> *(Ibid: 219).*

Introduction
Definitions of assessment
Assessment in the technical mode of practice
Assessment in the moral model of practice
Competence, a competency and competencies
Final comments
Further reading

Introduction

How formal summative assessment (the end of programme examination or other test) is presented within a teaching programme is crucial, because learners perceive the values behind that whole programme by analyzing what that final assessment requires of them. This tells them what matters to their teachers and the system. It teaches them what to focus on and what not to bother with. But there is more to assessment than this, and a far greater range of options available to the teacher.

Whichever mode of practice they work in, therefore, teachers have a solemn obligation to be clear about the implications of the assessment processes they use and about how to explain them to their learners. Where they work within the technical mode, teachers will, of course, construe assessment as the requirement to measure learners' outcomes in ways that have been set by a higher authority on behalf of whom they work. For those teaching in the moral mode and who are their own agents, there is both a responsibility to attend to the assessments set down in each learner's formal curriculum (to which they have an entitlement), and also to enrich that entitlement with assessment processes that they use additionally and which they design to support that learner's development (see chapter 11).

Thus, assessment can play very many different roles in different learning contexts. It can be used to keep a check on a learner's knowledge and understanding, as well as their performance and skills. It can be used to recognize and record their progress numerically, or to demonstrate their achievements over time. It can also be used to sort learners into categories for various purposes, though it cannot indicate exactly a learner's potential for the future. In much of this, assessment appears to rely on measuring the visible. But, it can also support the learner's on-going development — the development of personal attributes and character, and the development of the invisible drivers of practitioners' practice (like professional judgement or professionalism), as well of their developing wisdom. These are un-measurable, not being of the nature to be represented by numbers. They can, however, be 'evidenced' through the learner's words, which often provide richer details of developing understanding, offer the learner's own perspectives on their achievements, help teachers to understand 'where they are' in the learning process, and produce a record that learners can use as a base-line to establish their progress and that later teachers can easily understand and even re-evaluate.

Thus, arguably, there is a need in PGME to re-establish at minimum a balance between, on the one hand, seeing assessment simply as a technical process (a means of policing and measuring learning, of gate-keeping and of evaluating the success of the teaching), and on the other hand, seeing it as promoting learning, doing justice to its complexity, encouraging creativity and motivating the learner, as well as informing the teacher about the learner and their real needs, and feeding the learner's ability ultimately to self-assess.

This chapter is intended to contribute to what should be a debate at local and national level about the future purpose, design and use of assessment processes within PGME that are more educational than the current inaptly named 'Tools of the Trade'! The chapter also seeks to encourage teachers in PGME to become their own agents in respect of assessment — choosing their own view of it as a result of well-informed exploration, not merely accepting what has been imposed at national curriculum level. To these ends, various definitions of assessment are offered, followed by an overview of how assessment is seen first in the technical and then in the moral mode of practice. This leads on to a detailed look at competency-based and competence-based assessment. The chapter will end with a summary of assessment in the moral mode of practice.

Definitions of assessment

Definitions of assessment are directly linked to definitions of learning. Learning is seen by trainers as: *an outcome that is visible and measurable.* This 'outcomes' view is represented in the first (behaviourist) definition of learning found in chapter seven, Frame 7.1. By comparison, for educators, learning is about expanding and deepening understanding (see third definition in Frame 7.1). Here the implications are that assessment should have a far broader meaning, (See *Frame 8.1 A definition of assessment.)*

Frame 8.1 A definition of assessment

> Assessment is an all-embracing term. It covers any of the situations in which some aspect of a learner's education or training is in some sense measured/ recognized / or appreciated, whether this is by a teacher, an examiner or a learner themself. This process can be formal or informal. Broadly speaking it is concerned with demonstrating how well, and in what ways, a learner has profited (or is profiting) from the learning opportunities provided. But its educational value is ultimately governed by whether it was worth doing in the first place.

Assessment needs to be carefully distinguished from appraisal and evaluation. Assessment refers to learners' achievements. Appraisal is a system of exploring a professional employee's recent record in order to ensure that they are 'fit for purpose' within their institution and that they can fulfil the demands of their job. Once appraisals have been conducted over a set number of years, the evidence from them may then be used for revalidation of that individual as fit to be re-registered within their profession. Evaluation is about the quality of an educational or training *course or programme.* It should be noted that assessment (evidence of the quality of a learner's achievement) may be part of evidence used within both appraisal and evaluation processes, but it should not be confused with these processes and plays an equally important part in enabling the teacher to understand the learner's needs and achievements.

We often think of assessment as a formal process, but teachers make judgements about learners all the time (these are an *informal* form of assessment, but are often crucial for the student). Teachers therefore need to be vigilant about how and why they make them and, in order to be fair, such judgements must be principled, and the learners and all who receive the results of them should understand those principles. More about this can be found in chapter eleven, below.

Assessment in the technical mode of practice

The technical mode of practice, which is currently dominant in PGME, sees learning as about a change of behaviour (as gaining new skills and knowledge, or having the ability to pass an exam). In this view, the visible and measurable 'outcomes' of learning become the only evidence to be assessed, and are reported in terms of numbers. Providing numbers is assumed to give accurate and scientific evidence of the learner's achievement and this becomes the whole point of the training process. The end record of such assessment however, in leaving only numbers as concrete evidence, can be unsatisfactorily opaque in meaning to anyone viewing it at a later date. Further, as we shall see, the teacher's judgements inevitably come into play at all stages, thus introducing an inevitable subjectivity into the process!

Inside a system that chases qualifications for instrumental ends (see the box at the front of this chapter), this view of assessment becomes a goal in itself and leaves unchallenged its inaccurate assumption that assessment is an exact science. Postgraduate medical education, like almost all educational enterprises in the Western World, has been caught up into this psychometric approach to assessing learners. Indeed, it has become so prevalent that many do not even realize that there are other ways of seeing learning and learners and other ways of construing assessment. Ironically too, this notion that assessment is somehow scientific has caused a number of senior clinicians to engage in research projects seeking to perfect something that cannot be perfected, by trying to make this human system totally valid, reliable and accurate. See, for example: various attempts to quantify aspects of trainee surgeons' work (Kee et al. 1998; MacCormack and Parry 2006; Jacklin et al. 2008; Sevdalis and Jacklin 2008; Dijkstra et al. 2009).

It should not surprise us that no research team aiming to perfect the assessment of postgraduate doctors has yet reported the discovery of the unattainable nirvana they seek. Shocking though it may be for all those who are locked into seeing assessment this way, the fact is that they are trapped into a category mistake of assuming that everything that matters can be quantified, and so their endeavours will never provide a way forward. In this wonderland world, the improvement of assessment in PGME is seen as a technical problem in search of a technical solution. This lures the unwary to seek to measure the un-measurable and search for ways to introduce objectivity into a process that is inevitably and endemically subjective. It also blinds them to the other central component of assessment, which is the teacher's (or assessor's) professional judgement. (This is an important and valuable component and not the bugbear that technical rationalists see it as.)

Assessment then, is seen by most of those working in the technical mode of practice in PGME, as a *self-standing* enterprise that is the most central process of their work, and as essentially separate from teaching and learning. Indeed, for both trainers and those teachers who seek to inculcate their knowledge and skill into their learners and then look for them to regurgitate it, assessment is king. It provides the evidence of learning in a simple form, which is uncritically regarded as an indisputable guarantee that learning has happened (and that having happened, it will remain in place, unchallenged and unchanging). Assessment seen in this way also appears to enable teachers to demonstrate the absolute success of their teaching, thus making evaluation simple too!

All this arises from the seductive notion (unexamined and thus not critiqued) that assessment is the one element of teaching that is properly scientific, objective and therefore reliable, because it cashes out into numbers. This is what Broadfoot (2002) calls 'the myth of measurement', which she explodes as follows.

▷ Educational assessment can never be scientific.

▷ So-called psychometric tests can never be totally objective in the way that is claimed for them.

▷ The widespread acceptability of their significance 'lies not in their scientific worth, nor in the capacity of techniques developed to measure accurately what they purport to measure, *but quite simply because we believe in them*'. (italics mine)

(Summarized from *Broadfoot 2002: 215*).

Broadfoot's persuasive thesis is that the (unexamined) belief in the absolute accuracy of assessment rests on nothing more solid than the fact that the end result of assessment is reported in numbers. That the tyranny of the whole psychometric approach to assessment rests on such a fragile (indeed, mythical) basis is a very serious matter for our whole educational system. (See Broadfoot 2002: 203-230, but also, for example, Carr, D. 2003: 153-163.) This is especially so since a moment's thought about almost any assessment process which results in a very specific number, will be enough to recognize the blindingly obvious facts that: beneath its apparent objectivity there will always lie the subjectivity of the teacher's or assessor's judgement; that the result can never simply be the result of the straightforward application of some numerical scale; and that exact inter-rater reliability is, and always will be, an unachievable aim.

Further, this whole approach also engages trainers in some questionable logic, whereby assessment, being placed after the end of the teaching/learning event, fixes the entire aim for the whole event as: 'to produce evidence of a change in behaviour (or an exam pass)'. With this goal in view, the inevitable role of the trainer is to ensure that trainees can reproduce the required behaviour on demand, which means eschewing all else that might get in the way of that, however interesting or educational it might be. Such a narrow goal (with its manipulation of the learner and its ritualistic activities) seems unworthy of postgraduate education and of the intelligence of postgraduate doctors, and is unlikely to be *educationally worthwhile*. It is also a distortion of the educational processes of designing an educational programme and ignores the importance of educational aims (see chapter five above). This is because it banishes the unexpected and attends only to what has already been agenda-ed. It turns the process of teaching into a mere vehicle for 'delivering' an endpoint couched in figures, and renders the teaching process and the learner's product, un-motivating and unproductive, because they are not owned by those involved, having been predetermined by someone else. Thus, arguably, it distorts learning and teaching (see Carr, D. 2003: 155-64).

Postgraduate medical education was so besotted with this view of assessment (and its pseudo-science of 'objectivity, validity and reliability'), that, in 2002, when

I was asked by The Royal College of Surgeons of England to help them develop their first curriculum for surgical Senior House Officers, there was a universal (but unfulfilled) assumption that we would begin the whole curriculum design process by first formulating the assessments. Sadly, nearly ten years later, there is considerable evidence that nothing much has changed, despite the advent of curricula for all stages and specialties of PGME. This is mainly because, certainly in secondary care, a frightening number of clinical supervisors are still only dimly aware of the existence of the formal national assessment requirements, and beyond this, know even less about the formal Postgraduate Medical curriculum in their own specialty. However, those notable exceptions, whose educational understanding enables them to see through these assessment tools, are properly sceptical about their value. (See for example, Talbot (2004), whose title 'Monkey see, monkey do: a critique of the competency model in graduate medical education' aptly captures this view.)

Assessment in the moral mode of practice

By contrast to all this, for educators working in the moral mode of practice, assessment is a means of *promoting* learning, and is inextricably linked with teaching and learning and with learning about the learner. Indeed, assessment is a part of education, all of which is aimed at promoting and engaging the learner in *learning something appropriate to them, that is educationally worthwhile.* This means that assessment is in fact more complex than trainers recognize. It does not deliver absolute judgements on a learner's achievements and potential. But it offers a more honest and reliable, if less than totally specific, appreciation of the quality of the learner's achievements, based on evidence that is transparent and can be reviewed and considered both by those originally involved, and by others who work with the learner later along their educational pathway. Further, such evidence is in words, not in figures, and the words are the learner's own writing which gives direct evidence of their ability, rather than being presented in figures (or ticks on a list) chosen by the teacher as a label for the learner. (Practical details of this are offered below in chapter 12.)

Those who see themselves as involved in education rather than training, recognize assessment as complex and problematic because it is values-based. How we see the nature of assessment is shaped by how we construe learning and teaching and how we value assessment's processes and products. Further, there is no one means of assessment that will provide the whole picture of a person; of all that they can achieve; of all that they bring to their practice and of all that they have to offer as a professional. That is, there is no one single overall idea which will resolve all the conflicts within the decision-making about what to assess, how to assess it and what kind of evidence to seek. In fact we need a range of assessments (using different forms and from different perspectives) if we are to capture wide enough evidence to be able to talk realistically about the achievements of a human being. Yet assessment outcomes are so very powerful, that we treat the evidence from just one assessment event as quite unproblematic and as absolute, and definitive, such that people become unjustly labelled and then believe such labels! Worse, incomplete assessment of this kind provides information upon which many decisions are based, and has far-reaching effects — for individuals, for institutions, for the profession, and even for patients and the public.

In the moral mode of educational practice, a coherent *system* of assessment is seen as important because assessment crystallizes the whole process of education. This means that assessment is inextricably part of the related coherent processes of teaching and learning. Here, each choice made about assessment expresses a particular sense of educational purpose. Considered with all the parts of that process, each individual assessment event can give us useful information about ability and achievement. But even then we should treat it cautiously and certainly not use it as a label for life! A final assessment is never actually final, which is why the word 'summative' (meaning the summing up of what has been learnt so far), is more useful. Even then, our achievements may be radically reassessed and re-interpreted by someone who comes along later (either to our advantage or the reverse)!

If we do engage in assessment as a means of supporting teaching and learning and providing helpful information to teachers and learners *along the way*, then we can also with some confidence use the same results for *gate-keeping*, (the process of deciding whether to allow a learner to go through to the next level of career and of learning). Then we can be fairly sure that we have robust, extensive and detailed evidence to justify *professional* success or failure, and which is demonstrably fair and persuasive.

Assessment should not, therefore, be about pre-determined 'learning outcomes'. These should be treated with caution as no 'learning outcome' can be fully understood in isolation from the learner and the particular situation. The specific context of the learning and for the learner on that occasion, and the particular circumstances under which the 'outcome' was achieved, inevitably render it logically unable to be generalized. Yet one-off assessments are routinely treated as scientific and absolute! This is the reason why portfolios have become such popular means of collecting a wide range of evidence of our achievements. Their use shows that although assessment is often seen as related to tests and examinations, neither is essential to it. Further, as portfolios show, *assessment does not need to result in numbers or percentages.* If you are looking at patterns of a learner's achievement over time (which is what many portfolios do), then an overall classification of some kind (relating to broad grouping or levels) is more appropriate.

In the moral mode of practice, assessment is not just about looking at the visible surface of practice, but should plumb the depths of the professional values, thinking, character, decision-making and professional judgements of the learner. It should also take account of the person they bring to their practice of medicine (who meets the patient and cares for them). In this way we will be assessing what we have been teaching and the learner has been developing within the moral mode of practice. Thus, assessment is about:

- ▷ looking at the learner's achievements and progress *holistically*

- ▷ providing information that helps to shape further teaching and learning

- ▷ the learner's ability to learn

- ▷ the professional judgement of the teacher/assessor

- ▷ developing the learner's ability to self-assess

- ▷ how the learner has used the opportunities available for learning

- ▷ placing on record the learner's patterns of achievement, not using a one-off process to make decisions about a learner's future.

Some of these ideas also help us to distinguish between competency-based assessment and competence-based assessment. This is an important distinction that teachers in PGME need to be very clear about.

Competence, a competency and competencies

The differences of meanings between these three words are highly significant, have serious implications and account for many misunderstandings about assessment and medical curricula in general. This section will therefore offer some definitions, indicate the implications of the differences between competence and competencies, and explore each approach in detail.

Definitions

The word 'competence' is used to refer to an overall ability, at a required baseline standard, to meet all the demands of (in the case of medicine) being a fully professional doctor working in the service of patients at a particular level of post. This is not the same as 'expertise', which indicates a superior capacity to be aspired to, which good professionals strive for endlessly (because expertise is an open capacity that can never be totally mastered). Reaching competence does, however, indicate an acknowledgement that the doctor is fully equipped, *holistically*, to engage in medical practice. There is no such thing as a plural of this word. It is an overall term in itself (like 'education', where there is no plural because it is a comprehensive term in itself). This makes the NHS's habitual use of 'competences' in many of its documents very puzzling. At the point of obtaining recognition of competence, the doctor is declared 'competent' to work at that level (and therewith comes the reason for confusion between competent and competencies, as we shall now see).

The term 'competency' refers to one skill, and by grammatical logic, therefore (though not a logic that the NHS seems familiar with), the plural of that word is indeed, 'competencies' (like 'baby' and 'babies'). Thus, 'competencies' refers to a collection of skills. The word was first used in trying to list the skills that craftspersons or trade workers would need to learn to be able to do a job that required only the repetition of these skills in a given order and through a given method. Using this term to indicate that a doctor is ready to take up any post is therefore to short change patients. It indicates nothing more about the doctor than that they possess the sum total of skills necessary for that level. But practising medicine is not only about having skills (as we have seen). Further, overall competence in skills is more than about skills and involves more than the sum of individual skills learnt. The problem comes because it is perfectly possible to talk about being 'competent' in the skills learnt. Thus the same word is used, but means two very different things.

It should be noted that these days, where education for professional practice is construed within the technical mode, a 'competency-based curriculum' is the norm. Here the term competency is stretched to appear to cover every attribute a professional needs. This is inaccurate and inept. For example, how can professional judgement be 'a skill', how can 'being a caring doctor' be seriously reduced to a set of simple skills? What a distortion of professionalism this leads to when such attributes, capacities, professionalism and personal character are reduced to a series of simplistic items to be learnt through training. The competency-based curriculum (with its large lists of competencies to be mastered) lies at the centre of the technical mode of practice.

By contrast, an educational programme, referred to as a virtues-based curriculum, would resonate with the moral mode of practice. Here, whilst competencies (those skills and procedures that are central to medicine), together with theoretical knowledge, are still vitally important, there is more. Here the purpose of learning skills and knowledge is to use them in the service of patients as human beings. This emphasizes the importance of the quality of the doctor as a person, (and particularly as a morally focused professional) and also recognizes the invisible drivers of that doctor's conduct. A programme of professional education that nurtures growth in all these areas, at the same time as attending to the technical aspects of professional practice, would be based (as we have seen) on the Aristotelian virtues (and possibly also the Christian or other spiritual values). See The Appendix for a list of these.

Drawing the important distinctions

It is important to be clear about the contrast between competence and competencies. *Table 8.1 The vital distinction between competence and competencies*, illustrates this further. The first three paired cells on each side illustrate what has just been explained, the last five pairs explore the different language of 'capacities' and 'dispositions', and 'conduct' and 'behaviour'. The final paired cells demonstrate another way of expressing agency. The person who is holistically competent is shown as freely able to choose to exercise their capacity as appropriate and is open to being judged at the level of principle and intention. The person possessing competencies is shown as compelled by training to conform to outside standards of behaviour.

Table 8.1   The vital distinctions between competence and competencies

Competence: a holistic notion	Competencies: a number of skills
The term competent is used in both categories but means something very different in each	
Competent meaning: showing overall competence (including competencies).	**Competent** meaning: shows a competency and /or some competencies.
Eg: 'X is a wholly competent doctor'	Eg: 'This is a doctor whose competencies are signed off for his/her career stage.'
Meaning: 'X's overall competence shows as the ability to conduct him/herself and his/her work in different ways on different occasions according to what the situation demands (thus engaging in sound thinking) and *being* a good doctor as well as having the required skills and knowledge.	**Meaning:** this doctor has demonstrated the skills required and can use them as taught wherever s/he is required to perform or behave in this way. In this 'qualifying' process, emphasis has been placed on skills and knowledge. The person the doctor is has not been considered.
This is about **overall competence** – seen as holistic. This is a label for the **capacity** to operate reliable skills in a thoughtful manner.	This is about narrow atomistic skills, habits and mechanical efficiency. This is a label for **particular abilities** which are used unchangingly under all circumstances.
Here 'competent' means someone has: **a capacity** to operate successfully as a result of using their knowledge and skills flexibly (developed by education).	Here 'competent' means someone has: **a disposition** (has been shaped) to respond reliably and always in the same way (shaped by training or by being born thus).
Exercising a capacity means: a voluntary and deliberate exercise of principled judgement in the light of rational knowledge and understanding.	**Exercising a disposition** means: using inherent tendencies which enable agents to perform certain specifiable functions either through training or natural endowment.
Here the **competent** person is autonomous – a free agent whose aspiration/deliberate achievement is gained in the light of knowledge and professional standards.	Here the **competent** person has ability, power, effectiveness formed in him/her (by nature or training). Here competency has been instilled.
Here **conduct** is rationally ordered according to reason and principle.	Here **behaviour** is controlled by routine and reliability in the skills specified.
We choose to exercise our capacity. Here the *competent person is* acting in a broadly principled or reflective and informed way — and has to be judged on the basis of whether the principles were sound and the actions were moral and *achieved their intentions.*	Our dispositions exercise us (drive our actions). Here the **competent person** is acting well, efficiently and effectively according to some verifiable canon or acceptable standard of performance, which is the same for all circumstances.

(Adapted from Carr, D. 1993: 253-271)

The competency-based approach: nature and values

The skills-based approach to education for professional practice is based upon an unproblematic and simplistic view of the nature of professional practice, as something that has been sanitized of anything apparently subjective, including any moral dimension. It recognizes the need for professionals to be technically accountable, but, significantly, it does not value *moral answerability*.

This approach works by analyzing and listing what it deems as 'everything workers need to acquire in order to do their job'. It then categorizes all these items as either a competency or as knowledge. And all this it sees as able to be 'mastered'. This approach may work for simple routine jobs, and may improve some basic skills and even knowledge, quickly and visibly in the short term. But this 'atomising' approach to professional practice is unlikely to do justice to its complexity and further, in the longer term it may well create a rigidity of mind that is the opposite of the flexibility professionals need in their practice. It certainly has the advantage of being able to be readily organized into a bureaucratic model for administrative purposes, thus apparently increasing efficiency (and actually increasing bureaucratic control). It appears to lead to objective assessment of practice (though such apparent objectivity only hides further value judgements by the assessor). It is about improving visible, measurable performance (but often at the expense of understanding, personal development and all that underlies visible practice). It undervalues theory and research and has no interest in theorizing about practice or indeed in any theory that does not support behaviourism. It appears to seek scientific accuracy and objectivity and as such has no concept of or interest in the moral and ethical dimensions of professional practice.

The competency-based approach often does not offer professionals any inbuilt means of developing and refining their practice. It embraces the idea that professionalism can be judged only against the notion of fitness for purpose (but this ensures that the ends are never challenged). It emphasizes the acquisition of basic skills and knowledge but at the expense of developing understanding about how, where and when to use them, and is not interested in either refining further the practical and theoretical knowledge learnt, or in engaging in scholarly activity to develop them for the future. It is interested in behaviour that is visible (but not conduct which acknowledges the moral and ethical values, beliefs and theories which drive action). In short, it arises from a deficit model of professionalism, which believes that professional practice is the sum of a series of visible parts.

The competency-based approach values *certainties*. It teaches what it regards unproblematically as *the* knowledge, skills and strategies needed to be a successful professional. It values being able to analyze skills and the main observable characteristics of professional practice in the finest detail, and being able to measure these. It regards setting basic standards against which everything can be judged, as unproblematic and unquestionably objective, whereas these are notional and man-made constructs, created out of what is usually a political agenda. It regards training and measuring observable behaviour as a simple way of increasing efficiency. It is presented through the language and ideas of managerialism and of industrial output, which it regards as equally appropriate to discussing professionalism. In short, it is a model of 'how to work', which in no way recognizes the complexity of a professional's work.

The competence approach: nature and values

The competence approach to education for professional practice is based upon the view that professional practice is problematic and complex, being a human activity in which the nature of daily practice is uncertain, and a belief that it cannot therefore be aptly attended to via scientific processes. It sees such practice as a moral enterprise because professionals have a responsibility to vulnerable patients/clients, and colleagues. It recognizes the need for professional answerability in addition to their responsibility to be technically accountable.

This approach sees the work of professionals as involving open capacities that cannot be mastered. It recognizes the ability to utilize general knowledge, thinking and doing (which includes skills but far more) so that it is shaped to the specific and particular individual needs of patients. It emphasizes the importance of professional judgement and its complexity (the ability to choose between competing priorities, values, actions and interpretations). This brings with it the need to educate professionals to make wise choices in not only their main professional activities but also to understand the nature of different views of what constitutes education as an enterprise, and the implications of these. It sees education for professionals as focused on the development of a (personal) principled base from which to practise as a professional. In this, an understanding of the importance of values and self-knowledge in respect of the individual's professional values is important. Here there is a need to attend to the moral and ethical dimensions of practice.

Thus professionals need to develop the ability to consider their own progress by means of a range of approaches to assessment, which they have chosen rationally. This requires of the learner self-knowledge and the longer-term ability to attend to their own professional development. This too has wider implications. Professionals need to develop the ability to influence key decisions about assessment, how it is reported and the probity of its purposes, at the level of policy. This requires the capacity to take an active role in the development of assessment for the profession itself. One issue here may be about finding appropriate ways of placing on record an individual's understanding of the wider issues of professionalism and the responsibilities of being a member of a profession, because, for sure, the drive to *measure* professionalism springs from a category mistake, but this does not mean that professionalism cannot be evidenced in other ways (see Fish and de Cossart 2007. (These last two sub-sections have been adapted from de Cossart and Fish 2005.)

Final comments

If the learner should be a key agent in the learning process, as we said at the start of chapter six and argued throughout it, then there is need to integrate assessment with learning. Further, if formative (and to an extent, summative) assessment provides the teacher with understanding about the learner and their needs, then 'the ideal scenario would be to develop teaching and assessment strategies side by side' (Murphy 2002). In this view of practice in the moral mode, it would be illogical to conceive of assessment as a separate process, to design it without an eye on the learning processes and to expect teaching to be another separate activity. By contrast, in the technical mode of practice these processes are regrettably seen as separate.

Figure 8.1 Understanding Modes of Practice in Medical Education: the role of assessment, summarises the various relationships between teaching, learning and assessment as found in the technical and the moral modes of practice, by re-working Figure 3.1 as found at the end of chapter three. Here, the final face of each cube (now turned the other way in order that we can see a new face) is about assessment. Thus, for the narrowly technical mode, assessment dominates training and is used as a check on the end-product of learning through the learner's successful demonstration of the procedure, as trained — perhaps using a basic CBD, or DOPs or Mini-Clinical Examination (Mini-CEX). This does not prepare learners for the complexity of clinical practice (even within a 'real' procedure). In the full technical mode of practice, assessment uses all the 'Tools of the Trade' and the college examination of knowledge, again, to test or check on skills and knowledge, but focuses only on the visible aspects of practice and formal theory, which does not match the complexity of real practice.

By comparison, in the moral mode of practice assessment uses the 'Tools of the Trade' but supplements these with a range of other assessment processes that seek to attend to the invisible drivers of practice, to deepen the understanding behind the practice, and to nurture and develop the kind of person and professional the practitioner is. Here the focus is to prepare for the complexity of practice and to use assessment to promote learning.

Now see Figure 8.1 on the following page, where the key details of Figure 3.1 have been retained but new light brown flaps have been added to the boxes, that comment on the differing nature of assessment within each cube.

Figure 8.1 Understanding modes of practice in medical education: the role of assessment

(After the work of Carr, D. 2003)

(All modes may be needed but the educated teacher chooses them in an informed way)

Kind of professional	Highly restricted professional	Restricted professional	Extended professional
Kind of practitioner the teacher is	Working in the technical mode of practice	Working in the technical mode of practice	Working in the moral mode of practice

Extended professional

Medical teacher working in the moral mode of practice

concerned with **DEVELOPING conduct**

Holistic doctor

Uses and reflects on complex practice as main part of all assessment processes

A MORE COMPREHENSIVE ASSESSMENT in which the learner's knowledge, skills, character, capacities, professionalism, decision-making and judgement are uncovered in examples from real practice. Here assessment is employed to educationally worthwhile ends.

Restricted professional

Medical teacher working in the technical mode of practice

concerned with **SHAPING behaviour**

Technical doctor

Can pass 'Tools of the Trade' / exams: but not focused on real complex practice

A SIMPLE MATTER OF PASSING all tick-list assessments and exams. No real guarantee of ability in complex practice. No interest in harnessing assessment to promote learning.

Highly restricted professional

Technical trainer working in the technical mode of practice

concerned with **CHANGING behaviour**

all else irrelevant

little impact on practice

Technical trainee

Able to perform protocol OFTEN OUTSIDE REAL PRACTICE

A SIMPLE PROCESS, calling on *trained* skills that have been well learnt (uncritically) and observed by assessor watching performance and behaviour, but usually outside practice, applying rigid criteria which do not promote wider education

Assessment

Kind of learner

Assessment details

This chapter, then, has sought to equip PGME teachers with a grasp of the short- and long-term implications of the distinctions between these two views, thereby enabling them to articulate their own position on the assessment of postgraduate doctors. For those who wish to engage in the creative processes of enriching the required technical processes of assessment, chapters 11 and 12 below will offer a range of practical ideas.

Indeed, it is now time to turn from our attempt in Part One to clarify a series of matters related to *thinking like an educator*, and to consider the practical implications of all this, which is the focus of Part Two.

Further reading

* Talbot, M. (2004) 'Monkey see, monkey do: a critique of the competency model in graduate medical education', *Medical education*: June **38** (6): 587-92.

Carr, D. (1993) Questions of Competence, *British Journal of Educational Studies*, **41**: 253-271.

Part Two

The practical implications:

how changing understanding changes practice

Chapter Nine

Enriched teaching in medical practice: towards *praxis*

> I did train... I now teach... but most excitingly, next I want to ... strive to achieve educational *praxis*.
>
> .... I aspire to be an enhanced teacher, one who engages learners before, during and after the teaching event. I will recognise the complexities involved in the practice of education (and clinical practice) and be curious about my own practices. I will inspire learners to become independent thinkers and thus creators of new practice, who will take on the development of their profession.
>
> Extract from the educational philosophy
> of one of the PG Cert members
> referred to in chapter one.

Introduction
Responsibilities and definitions
Thinking like an educator: planning for teaching
Thinking like an educator: methods and content, evaluation and quality
Developing your own educational philosophy

Introduction

Part One of this book has argued for PGME to be refocused from its present all-consumingly narrow technical concerns towards the wider moral mode of practice. This is the case, not only for the practice of teaching but also for the practice of medicine. Such a view demands a reshaping of the responsibilities of PGME teachers, requiring them both to adopt new approaches to education and also to enable the doctors who learn from them to set the technical aspects of medical practice into a wider view of their professional responsibilities. To this end, it was argued, such teachers should aspire to be educators who engage in educational *praxis* — to become advanced teachers who act as educators. Such teachers provide what is educationally worthwhile for each learner, actively develop a refined educational judgement, make wise selections from a range of *educational principles*, and use these wisely within practice.

The four chapters in Part Two now seek to illustrate the thinking that informs wise educational practice and which advanced teachers should engage in. Chapter nine looks at this *from the teacher's point of view*. It focuses on ways of thinking about one's own teaching by highlighting some key principles of planning that underlie *praxis* (where the teacher seeks to engage in morally shaped action). It also demonstrates how the teacher with a disposition to act wisely can prepare for, and think educationally about, each learning event, harnessing practical reasoning to ethical ends. Subsequent chapters in Part Two then focus in similar ways on the learner and on informal and formal assessment.

Those who are disappointed that Part Two does not list simple teaching skills, strategies and tips for teachers, are reminded of the lesser role that technical matters play in the moral mode of practice. Readers seeking more technical advice are referred to the many books offering tips for teachers, managerial strategies and theories from domains like psychology and sociology (see, for example, Dornan, Mann, Scherpbier and Spencer 2011). In the eyes of those practising teachers *who are educators by profession,* however, such texts are not seen as exploring the real richness and substance of education *as a professional practice.* The contribution of such publications may well be to remind would-be teachers of some basic skills and strategies or even some generalized theory that might offer them some technical support. But by atomizing teaching as a set of technical skills and knowledge to be applied more or less randomly to teaching events, such publications do not characterize fully the real educational enterprise.

Indeed, as previously noted, pp. 87-8, where educationally worthwhile learning has been achieved, the teacher can claim to have been an educator, irrespective of their educational 'know-how' or skills. Further, where the experience has not been educational, no amount of teaching skills will compensate, and no technical know-how will make the experience educational for learners, (see Carr, W. 1995:160). That is why what is offered here are principles and ideas to fuel a teacher's thinking about their educational practice. Principles are not rules and cannot be reduced to practical tips. Rather they encourage personal decisions about how to enact these principles and which to emphasize.

As a basis for what follows then, this chapter begins by defining the overall and the specific responsibilities of PGME teachers and offering some important definitions. Useful principles and practical examples then follow in relation to: thinking like an educator; planning for, preparing, and engaging in teaching within the moral mode of practice; and developing your own educational philosophy by exploring your educational values.

Responsibilities and definitions

The GMC has long since defined the very basic requirements and responsibilities for engaging in postgraduate teaching in medical practice. Ideas about what is involved in 'good' teaching are, as we have seen, dependent on one's educational values, and until now the very basic technical approach to teaching has determined the definitions and expectations of PGME. What follows offers a contrasting view, which comes from the moral mode of practice, of firstly the overall responsibilities of the advanced teacher and then of the specific roles of the educational and clinical supervisor. This is followed by a clear indication of what is meant in this book by the 'good' and 'wise' teacher.

Overall responsibilities for PGME teachers

An advanced educator in PGME has a responsibility to see education as a holistic enterprise and to treat their learners as whole persons. They are also the designers of the education they offer, being their own agents and mediating the formal curriculum to suit the individual needs of their learners and those learners' patients. They have a vision of education as having coherence, continuity, and cohesion, and they seek to link all the elements they offer into an ever spiralling coalescence that educates the doctor holistically, and looks towards their longer-term education throughout their career — all of which conduces to safer and better patient care.

To this end such teachers also have a responsibility to develop themselves as people who are more perceptively and affectively attuned to their educational responsibilities to cultivate their learner ontologically (as a person) as well as epistemologically (in terms of knowledge, and skills). Thus, they bring their own human and clinical experience to attend to the learner's developing conduct and personhood and are responsible for providing education that is finely adjusted to each learner's needs, and for supporting and challenging learners to aspire to greater achievements, including increasingly thoughtful clinical practice.

Education is focused on the pursuit by *teacher and learner* of virtues rather than competencies, on the human not merely the technical. In this view, it is not the possession of teaching methods and skills that determine the successful teacher, but the quality of person the teacher is. The Appendix offers several ways of expressing the virtues, and shows that although they are based on different values (classical and Christian) such ideals are generally accepted as the basis of good conduct and have been so in most parts of the world for many centuries.

Teaching has a rich tradition as a practice within which a teachers' moral and intellectual understandings are derived from *within themselves* as teachers, not by being the agent of another. Teaching as a practice has its own integrity — to those who are thoughtful about what they do as teachers. This is why our deepest responsibility is, as Hansen argues, that we should first determine what we care about as morally responsible teachers [of postgraduate doctors] 'and then craft a conception of teaching that coheres with that determination' (Hansen 2001: 4). In this, the list of virtues might offer a starting point for discussion!

Given the extreme pressures on clinical practice, PGME educators also have the important responsibility to fight for respect from colleagues and managers for the educational enterprise itself and for privileging appropriate times and places within which it should happen. They also need to establish for themselves and with their colleagues the recognition of a moral obligation to use the learner's time as educationally soundly as possible and to honour it as much as they prize working with patients. This requires a clear view of the main educational achievements that can and should arise from working with that learner educationally (clarity about aims and their rationale), and the setting up of activities such that other, unexpected, educational benefits may also occur and prove seriously enlightening, on the day.

The differing responsibilities of clinical and educational supervisors

An analysis of the educational responsibilities that PGME undertakes for learning doctors shows the following four main areas of activity.

1. **The formal educational programme.** This is set within a Trust department and aimed at providing lectures, presentations and group learning. This is often addressed by a variety of 'inputs' on special topics by a wider range of presenters, but it may or may not be immediately relevant to the learning doctor's individual needs in being a practising clinician. Further, the quality of the teaching offered may be variable and is likely to have been conceived as a one-off activity by the presenter. A better way to use this time might be group discussion of cases and procedures, table-top ward rounds and other ways of probing and developing learners' thinking.

2. **The educational/managerial overview.** Here the educational supervisor oversees the doctor's learning within a post or programme (where the doctor's overall educational progress is attended to).

3. **Privileged educational interactions in or near the clinical setting.** These develop the doctor educationally as a person and a clinician on a regular basis. This is where the doctor's main educational needs are attended to directly by their clinical supervisor, guided by the relevant curriculum. This is the element that is currently often submerged into the fourth and final category, but ironically is the most important educationally!

4. **Continuous daily clinical supervision.** Here, the doctor as a clinician is *supervised clinically* by their clinical supervisor as they work with and for patients in the clinical setting. The supervisor's key role is to oversee the learning doctor's clinical actions, decisions, thinking, and patient management, primarily assuring the safe care of patients. Alertness to diagnosing that doctor's learning needs, as shown up in their practice, and/or to spotting key learning opportunities in what occurs, is also important but is secondary to patient safety and optimal care. Thus the issues that clinical supervisors highlight in practice need to be attended to in 3. above.

The main purpose of these definitions is to be clear as to what is a general programme of presentations for a learner, what is a full educational interaction with a learner and what is primarily a clinical interaction which may be educational at a secondary level or may reveal a learning need to be attended to later. Where this distinction is not clear, learning doctors who may have the wrong expectations of an event which is primarily clinical supervision, may feel (unjustly) that their education has not been attended to, and that what they have been offered is not 'educationally worthwhile'.

What does 'educationally worthwhile' teaching mean?

For the purpose of discussing these matters, in order to provoke debate, and to generate more broadly-based understanding of education as a practice in PGME, the term 'educationally worthwhile' as used in relation to teaching doctors in the clinical setting, is taken to mean as follows. See *Frame 9.1 PGME that is 'educationally worthwhile'*.

Frame 9.1 PGME that is 'educationally worthwhile'

> PGME that is educationally worthwhile is the practice of teaching as shaped by the overall aim of using wisely in an educationally-informed way and for appropriate purposes, the most precious time in which teacher and learner meet together. To this end the preparation for, engagement with and follow-up from this learning event will be guided by generally accepted sound educational principles. It also assumes that each teaching/learning event is part of an overall educational enterprise in which teachers take every learning opportunity to engage the doctor as a whole person and to attend holistically to their education as appropriate, given their needs, post, curriculum and seniority.
>
> The educationally worthwhile results from educationally well-informed decisions and properly formulated educational aims, having reviewed a range of possibilities available, about what content as well as which teaching, learning and assessment processes are best to use in working with this particular learner in this particular context, in order to maximize that learner's improvement and achievements as a person and a doctor.

Some things can be learnt without the teacher being there, though these may need to be reviewed with the learner. But the most valuable (educationally worthwhile) intentions, for the teacher working with an individual postgraduate doctor, are achieved when the learner and the teacher engage together to well-directed ends. Such intentions need to take account of the learner's curriculum requirements but should not be trammelled by them. The best intentions will emerge from exploring the learner's needs, interests, starting points and appropriate aspirations, from the perspective of the moral mode of medical practice and the needs of that doctor's current patients. As we said above pp. 95-6 it is important here to distinguish between the learner's wants and needs (see Wilson 1971). The resulting intentions should be crystallized in writing and refined *with* the learner.

Behind these intentions lies an aim that captures an even deeper moral responsibility — that of improving the quality and safety of patient care. Doctors who know more and who understand that knowledge better, who have greater skill, whose clinical judgements are increasingly wise and whose expertise is shaped also by knowing *who they are* as doctors and human beings, will be best placed to work more expertly with patients.

'Good' and 'wise' teaching

In order to discuss the attributes of sound practical teaching and how to strive to achieve and improve these, we need to make clear the meaning of the words 'good' and 'wise' as used here. Such words are values-based and can mean different things depending on which approach to teaching one espouses. The following offers a careful stipulative definition of each as used in this book and indicates how this usage relates to more common uses of the word.

So, what is 'good' teaching?

The word 'good' is broadly used as an accolade and indicates approval. For our purposes, to label an action or activity 'good', indicates that it is *a virtue in itself* — and thus an end in itself. This means that the activity is not carried out for an ulterior motive! When attached to the word 'teaching', it also indicates that 'good' is the goal for the practice of teaching. That is: 'Good' teaching is a means to 'good ends', (a learner who has gained valuable and worthwhile things, like understanding and knowledge). Thus, in the moral mode of practice, good teaching is a virtue in itself.

In the technical mode of practice good teaching would be about having the right kind and number of teaching competencies (as decreed by some national body). Good teaching in schools is currently standardized against such a list, but the unlooked-for results of this are beginning to emerge as boredom suffered by both teachers and learners who are required to be the passive agents of the curriculum, rendering them unimaginative and uncreative. By contrast, the term, *good* teaching as used in this book, refers to: 'the possession and exercise by the teacher of a range of virtues of a broadly Aristotelian kind, including practical wisdom *(phronesis)'* (Dunne and Hogan 2004: xviii). This is about making wise and morally sound judgements. It should be noted that these spring from the character rather than the technical proficiency of a good teacher. Thus, a good teacher is good more because s/he is a good person who also promotes educationally worthwhile learning, than because s/he possesses a given number of organizational skills and teaching strategies.

Thus, good teaching is not about good performance but is more about good personhood that drives a moral awareness and a moral mode of engagement with learners. Because teaching therefore has an inextinguishably moral dimension, in seeking to become a good teacher one is called to personal transformation of heart and soul. (See Carr, D. 2007.)

Being a 'wise' teacher who exercises phronesis

Being a 'wise' teacher who exercises *phronesis*, in this context picks up Aristotle's meaning of wise, and is used particularly in respect of judgement. Wisdom in working like this takes time to develop but it does provide an ideal to aspire to (and sometimes to reach). Such an approach to education involves the teacher in a commitment to each learner, which (though not limitless) certainly involves active concern, a will to work with rather than on the learner, and a kind of open-ended helpfulness and perhaps intelligent kindness. This requires achieving a balance of commitment to one learner, with one's responsibility to all other learners, and (in medical education) to the best interests of patients. At the heart of being a wise teacher are both the motivations and ethical principles that each teacher brings as a professional educator, to recognize, navigate through and resolve (temporarily), the ambiguities inherent in 'serving the learner'.

Thinking like an educator: planning for teaching

This section first offers some important principles for developing educationally worthwhile teaching, considers some questions about educational aims and then provides a range of important questions that a teacher needs to consider in order to prepare properly for and engage fully in educationally worthwhile teaching.

Some principles for providing educationally worthwhile teaching of postgraduate doctors

Eight key principles offer a sound basis for preparing for and conducting worthwhile education. They are as follows.

1. Educational aims and specific intentions must come first in a teacher's thinking if the enterprise is to be counted as education. The choice will depend on one's values. These should be considered before all other decisions about how to teach, learn, assess, and evaluate. (See Part One, p. 82.)

2. Sound and meticulous planning for teaching and learning is absolutely essential. Good preparation is the hallmark of quality teaching. The main focus of educationally worthwhile planning in PGME should be about developing, sharpening and critiquing the learner's being, knowing, doing, thinking and becoming, in respect of their medical practice as a doctor. This is about developing conduct, not changing behaviour. It should seek to improve clinical understanding, which goes beyond mere knowledge of the required facts and which informs good clinical judgement, and this should promote improved clinical practice and better patient care. (See Part One, pp. 52,64,79.)

3. In order to offer educationally worthwhile teaching it is necessary to study the learner and the learner's needs and interests as a developing doctor, and recognize the teacher's responsibility to attend to that learner by meeting them as a person who has personal and professional values and aspirations. Educationally worthwhile teaching is, by definition, based on sound educational relationships between teacher and learner. (See Part One, p. 97.)

4. Teaching should, however also be construed as an enterprise in which the teacher and learner think and act together creatively towards ends, only some of which are pre-designed. (See Part One, p. 88.)

5. Full interaction with learners in a detailed professional conversation will frequently need to be adopted as it is a key vehicle for education, which leads naturally to the teacher needing to develop a range of expertise in language in order to promote thinking (as opposed merely to promoting description and narrative in learners). (See Part One, pp. 93-4.)

6. Learners should be supported and guided by teachers to engage in reflection on their own professional and clinical experiences so as to make clinically sound meaning out of them. (See Part One, pp. 115-17.)

7. Resource-based learning is the centre of this approach to education, in which the learner does much of the work and the teacher, as an expert in a range of language strategies, promotes deeper thinking in the learner. (See Part One, p. 97.)

8. The basis of such teaching is the development of a personal educational philosophy or credo in respect of what is involved in enriched and advanced teaching. (See Part One, pp. 35,79.)

Of these principles, 3, 5, 6, and 7 will shape the content of chapter ten below, while this chapter concentrates on the rest.

Thinking about aims and intentions

Whilst the wider educational aims of a teaching programme are usually pre-set, a teacher can critique these, interpret them in a range of ways and then set their own intentions for their own teaching sessions. This section offers a range of issues about which a teacher needs to think carefully in setting intentions for their for teaching. Such thinking cannot be done by someone else and it needs fresh re-consideration for each new learner. (See chapter five above.)

When we seek to express educational intentions we find the following sorts of phrases occurring to us, but we need to monitor these carefully since each carries a particular nuance. For example:

▷ promote the growth of understanding or intellectual enquiry

▷ develop potentialities to the full or all-round ability

▷ consider the needs of society, in stressing art, culture, moral issues

▷ encourage flexibility, creativity, imagination, rationality, benevolence, tolerance

▷ cultivate intellect, skill, knowledge

▷ shape character, conduct, judgement, criticality

▷ emphasize specialisms

▷ inculcate culture and tradition

▷ prepare the learner for joining a particular part of society

▷ ensure that standards of professionalism are adhered to.

Thus, as discussed in chapter five, aims and intentions are based within certain metaphors. In the biological model of education, *nature* is the core and *growth* is the metaphor (see the first five items in the above list). Here education is a process of growth or development towards a final end, it is the cultivation of individuality, of self-realization, and of the fullest development of one's potential, which the teacher encourages. For many (if not most) PGME teachers their intentions will surely include developing moral dispositions. Overdone, however, this can be so learner-centred that teachers make no interventions at all. (See Part One p. 85.)

The approach that is traditionally contrasted with this is the model of education in which *nurture* is the core and *initiation* is the metaphor (see the second five in the list above). Here, education is a social enterprise and rules are agreed as the product of a society or culture and must be learnt so that tradition is maintained. But, overdone, this can unreasonably promote particular views and values. (See also Part One, p. 85.)

It will be clear, in the light of this that balances needs to be kept and care needs to be taken in expressing intentions. The educator's job in PGME may be both to encourage growth in the learner and to initiate them into the traditions of their profession. They may need to enlighten understanding (so that learners know enough to make sound choices) and to develop dispositions (courage, patience, strength, reflection, to act wisely). Further, some intentions are deeply related to others — for example the twin intentions of helping the learner to possess knowledge and understanding, and to develop the necessary dispositions to use this wisely are interwoven (the educated learner can't have one without the other). Some intentions, however, may be contradictory!

Further, in deciding what educational intentions should direct our work, we need to remember not to restrict learning to those matters that we are aware of before we start to teach. Teaching/learning should be creative and lead to the discovery of new and unexpected learning outcomes as well as those predicted. We should treasure the unexpected, providing it is educationally appropriate.

Planning and preparing for teaching in the moral mode of practice

Frame 9.2 Some important issues for planning offers what, the teacher must think carefully about, choose appropriately from, and find ways of dealing with or discovering more about, in order to be a successful *educator*.

Frame 9.2: Some important issues for planning

> The teacher needs to think about the following at specific stages in planning to teach.
>
> 1. In preparation for being an advanced teacher in the clinical setting

What sort of professional do I value and want to develop?
What are my learner's views on this?
What ideas about teaching and learning do I value?
What are my learner's views on this?
What does my profession and specialty value?
What do I want any learner to achieve broadly as we work together?

2. At the beginning of arranging to work with a learner
What kind of practitioner does this learner want to be?
What are the curriculum requirements for the learner & this attachment?
What are the learner's intentions and needs for this attachment?
Are they appropriate?
What can this attachment offer / what can the whole department offer?
What are the formal educational intentions for this programme?
Are they are understood by both teacher and learner?
What else might be useful to teach beyond these basics?
What should be the key intentions for this learner in this attachment?

3. When planning for a specific teaching session
How should we decide what the learner would focus on in this session?
How do I know what the learner needs in this session?
What is the learner's starting point for all this?
What is the level of the learner's motivation and incentive to learn this?
What is the central nature of what the learner needs to learn here?
Which matters associated with the moral mode of practice need attention?
In what setting should this session take place?
Given what I know of the learner, what is the best approach to this?
What are the best educational methods / broad strategies to use here?
How will I ensure we engage in sound educational interaction?
What do we need to do to prepare for and to follow up on this session?
Is there any self-directed learning the learner can engage in?
How am I going to start and what will be the logic of the structure of the taught session?
What key educational judgements am I likely to have to make?
What would count for success in this learning?
What should the teacher do and what should the learner do to achieve this?
What key activities should the learner engage in? (new learning/revision/creativity/ look at old material in new ways?)
Over what period does this need to happen?
What resources will need to be supplied /collected (how will I ensure their appropriateness)?
How might new and creative issues emerge during the session?
What might the learner achieve: how will this relate to the intentions?
What will be the evidence of the learner's achievements?

What will be a good way to record this evidence?

How can the *learner* do that recording?

What follow-up will embed, sustain and extend this educationally worthwhile learning?

What will we reflect on afterwards and to what ends?

How will we evaluate it all?

Sound planning (thinking) at the early stage is essential in shaping worthwhile education. The above checklist can be used as a guide in both setting the learning contract for the whole programme of the attachment and in preparing for a smaller educational sequence within it. However, it should be used as a guide and not a protocol.

Thinking like an educator: methods and content, evaluation and quality

We have already indicated the range of influences that should be considered in thinking about what to teach a given learner. This section will take this further by exploring six significant issues already highlighted in Part One:

▷ the importance of focusing on the ordinary rather than the extra-ordinary as found in the clinical setting

▷ the usefulness of three curriculum models that help the teacher see different ways of engaging in teaching

▷ the importance of differentiation as a principle that ensures all learners in a group gain educationally from the teaching

▷ the teaching of a procedure so that it can be more than just training in the process

▷ the significance of the tacit professional judgements that the teacher makes during a teaching session in order to orchestrate the various elements that conduce to on-the-spot learning

▷ the benefits of reflective evaluation on the teaching/learning process.

Teaching the ordinary

In very properly using the clinical setting itself as a resource, clinicians often turn to focus on the dramatic — on complaints or critical events — as a means to their educational ends. But clinician-teachers really need to maximize learning from all that happens. It is arguable that the core of good clinical teaching (supervision) should actually be 'ordinary practice' and everything else should be conceived of as around that core. After all, everyday events, being ninety per cent of clinical practice are therefore ninety per cent of what the learner needs to learn from PGME. Clinical teachers should not concentrate on things that go wrong to the neglect of the things that they do daily.

Perhaps rather, the springboard of PGME teaching should be those *important but taken-for-granted ordinary events of clinical practice* (about the practice of patient care and the effectiveness of doctors as clinicians). This means the teacher first unpacking their own invisible thinking and knowing both during moments of their own clinical activity and during moments of pause or silence while waiting for the next piece of action. For example it is possible to:

▷ think aloud and give a running commentary – especially in moments of pause / silence / waiting, as well as during key activities

▷ play the 'what if it was different in this way' game

▷ send learner out to investigate something relevant and report back

▷ set the learner up to keep a log during the clinical session of some key issue

▷ equip the learner with a list of things to be looking for or thinking about (that will be discussed afterwards).

All this can make teaching during 'ordinary clinical practice' more overtly educational.

Three models of teaching

As noted in Part One, pp. 108-9, Stenhouse (1975) offers us three different models to aid the teacher's thinking about how to go about such teaching. His work conceptualized the relationship of teaching, learning and assessment as concerned with different educational models or mind-sets about teaching: the product, the process and the research model. However, such models should be used wisely by the teacher to help consider the whole educational enterprise, and not be taken as exclusive approaches to adopt wholesale in teaching.

The greatest value of Stenhouse's work is in the way it captures three different mindsets about education, in which the values and assumptions about the role of the teacher, the learner and assessment are all very different (see *Table 9.1 Three Models of Teaching*). This shows that the logic of each is self-contained and separate from the others. This table was originally made public in Fish and Coles (2005).

Table 9.1 Three Models of Teaching

Education as a product	Education as a process	Education as research
Intention		
teacher transmits knowledge	teacher promotes knowledge	learner explores understanding
Locus of knowledge		
resides in teacher	resides in teachers & learners	resides in learner group
Student activities		
passive learners	active learners	aware of selves as active learners and negotiators
(covers material fast)	(active learning takes longer)	(this takes even longer)
Motivation via		
teacher	own active learning	group learning / active learning
Sees learner as		
receiver of knowledge	active seeker of knowledge	discoverer / reconstructor of own knowledge
Sees teacher as		
teller / instructor	seeker / catalyst	facilitator / neutral chair
Teaching activities		
presenter/ lecturer	facilitates learning, sets up problems, probably knows answers	teacher is leader within group but learns alongside them
Sees assessment as		
end of course tests, summative, teacher assessment	part of teaching, part of learning, formative - and summative	self-assessment, group assessment, aiding understanding
Plans by means of		
aims; objectives; content; summative assessment	aims; intentions; list of content; assessment as part of this process	aims; intentions; counselling-type methods; assessment within this process
Use of resources		
chosen by teacher and brought into the learner's context from outside by the teacher, and thus may not relate to learner's context.	learner-centred and thus inevitably arising from the learner's context and relevant to it.	learner organized and thus chosen from the learners' context
View of professional		
teacher is a performer whose performance is significant in the quality of learners' education	teacher as facilitator sets up learning for learners and teacher's input features less in the sessions	teacher as facilitator learns alongside learners, but this can only be on a highly disciplined basis

Thus, in the **Product Model**, where knowledge is seen as a package that the learner is to come to possess, the teacher's role is to provide this by transmission, the learner is seen as a passive receiver of this and is then tested to check that the transaction has properly taken place. Everything else then follows from this in terms of the roles of teacher and learner, the motivation, and the resources and their use. By contrast, the **Process Model** sees teaching as an exploratory process that rests on interaction between the teacher and the learner, where the aim is to help the learner to seek understanding and to make it their own by working with it actively. Thus the roles of teacher and learner are more collaborative, learning is active, and assessment during the learning helps both teacher and learner to see current achievements and also to readjust the processes of teaching and learning. In the third model, the **Research Model**, education is characterized as research-based and the aim is about enabling learners to explore understanding and to become emancipated from knowledge 'handed down' to them. Here, they both learn, and also exercise their critical faculties in relating it to their current understanding by investigating issues for themselves under the teacher's guidance. In this model, the roles of teacher and learner become genuinely collaborative and investigative; assessment takes its part fully in the teaching and learning process, and itself is driven collaboratively; and the context becomes central, as the place in which education takes place. Thus, each model leads to a different kind of educational achievement for the learner, each prioritizes different intentions, and each also sees teaching, learning and assessment in a different temporal relationship. Each therefore has a role to play in education.

As well as considering this range of overall educational models in thinking about how to proceed as a teacher, it is also necessary to be aware of the different impact of teaching on different learners, such that where there are several learners in one teaching session together, they may need different attention. In the teaching profession providing for this is called 'differentiation'.

The importance of 'differentiation'

'Differentiation' is a teaching term which indicates that, within any group of learners who are working together there will be different levels of experience or ability. The teacher should therefore adjust task and/or level of challenge for each learner to take account of each individual's ability, while also maintaining a group approach to the topic, where possible using each learner as a resource for the others, and encouraging all to aspire to their best.

In PGME, where more than one learner is present in the discussion with the consultant, it is likely that such learners will also be at very different career stages. Thus, their varying experience needs to be carefully taken into account so that, while all are contributing to a group focus, and will teach and learn from each other, the tasks they will prepare privately are properly *differentiated* across learners in relation to their different career stage and individual ability. See particularly Fish and de Cossart (2007:137- 42) where an example of this is demonstrated.

Differentiation then is one example of wise educational judgement by the teacher that ensures that learners are experiencing educationally worthwhile learning. Here, judgement needs to be made both during planning for teaching and also whenever the teacher needs to adjust pace, timing and content during the teaching session.

Re-conceiving the teaching of a procedure as an educational rather than merely a training activity also requires such judgement.

How the teaching of a procedure should involve more than just training in the process

Table 9.2 *Teaching a procedure: turning training into education*, offers an illustrative example of how teaching a procedure can be transformed by teaching in the moral mode of practice. This Table was first published in Fish 2010: 200-01.

Table 9.2 Teaching a procedure: turning training into education

The training plan to teach a procedure	The educational plan to teach a procedure
Aim: To inculcate in the learner the ability to do X as a professional doctor/ healthcare practitioner.	*Aim:* To enable the learner to do X and develop the abilities of doing, thinking, knowing and critiquing the doing of X as a professional doctor/healthcare practitioner.
To steep the learner in technical rational ways of thinking about and engaging in practice, which creates a rule-following mindset, and absolves the practitioner from taking moral responsibility for individual cases.	To introduce explicitly the practical reasoning required of a clinical practitioner, and develop a mindset that expects to call upon and be able to articulate the professional judgments made in individual cases.
Objectives or learning outcomes:	*Intentions:*
	To enable learners to:
By the end of the training the learner will be able to do all the subdivisions of action involved in X procedure, and string them together as a routine.	• learn how to do X as a whole procedure • explore the *thinking/knowing/doing/being* that they engage in as they do this procedure well (by doing and reflecting in detail each time)
To generate evidence of the learner's ability to do this by giving an acceptable performance that achieves the end this procedure is designed to bring about.	• consider the implications of doing X under various conditions • discover the strategies they need to use in a variety of different patient cases • understand what is involved for each individual patient • explore critically the wider uses of procedure X • understand the issues raised by doing procedure X • self-assess the quality of their doing X.

Teaching methods (emphasis on teacher)	*Teaching methods* (emphasis on learner)
Teacher informs, instructs, demonstrates, but has little idea what the learner understands, knows, and thinks.	Learners develop their own skills, as appropriate and *make their own* the language, concepts, and knowledge of the teacher. These seem slower at first but lay the basis for safe practice that will never require basic revision.
These seem to provide a quick fix at the start. But this approach is potentially dangerous for patients and disconcerting for learners, who often later run into events they are not equipped for.	1. Get learner to *prepare for doing this procedure*. (What does that involve for *this* learner and *this* procedure?) 2. Prepare as teacher for this learner and this patient. (What does this involve on this occasion?)
3. Demonstrate X by performing all the actions involved and giving a commentary. Demonstrate a second time, asking learner to provide a running commentary.	3. Engage learner in understanding what is involved in the activity of doing X (demonstrate /talk together).
	4. Reflect: Either have a conversation about what learner gained from the observation, or get learner to write a bit about what they gained from it. 5. Raise issues about when, where and why to do X (or not), so that learner sees the wider professional and medical issues.
6. Ask learner to do X while you provide a commentary. Tell learner to do X and to provide a running commentary.	6. Get learner to do a simple example of X. 7. Reflect afterwards with learner (in dialogue) about the *being/thinking/ knowing/doing* involved. Encourage learner to articulate own strategies, ways through, ways of understanding what s/he is doing. *Assess formatively.* 8. Get learner to write about that experience, to explore this further and crystallize own version. Then respond to this briefly in writing. *Add to this one event, a number of the same.* 9. Ensure that learner can provide *all* the patient care necessary for the whole procedure from preparation to follow-up. 10. Let learner do a range of cases. Talk with the learner as s/he works, using a collaborative dialogue. 11. Engage the learner in further exploration/ reflection/reading.

12. Assess performance of what has just been practised. This is summative. This changes behaviour quite quickly but it may only be changed while the learner is being watched.	12. Run a summative assessment of the entire process and procedure as completed in real practice, and document accordingly. This changes understanding, which takes longer. But it thus becomes *conduct* that you can count on, because it is informed behaviour.
Here, teaching itself is perceived as a technical rational activity in which teaching is seen as a performance and the invariable rules are set out for the teacher as well as the learner, in clearly instructional terms and in a required order (informed by behavioural psychology).	Here, teaching is perceived as an activity informed by practical reasoning, where only the principles that guide the teaching are set out, and the teacher makes decisions about how to adapt these to the context. Imaginative and inspirational teaching is developed rather than instructed (Carr, D. 2000: 8), and engages the learner in resource-based learning.

As will quickly be evident, both processes attend thoroughly to learning to do the procedure but the educational process which is seated in the moral mode of practice is conceived quite differently from the training or technical approach. Each is shaped by different aims followed by objectives for training, and by intentions for education, while the training approach calls for far fewer steps and conceives of assessment differently.

This particular example shows very clearly the differences between teaching in the two different modes of practice. It will be an educational judgement on the part of the teacher as to whether or not working in the moral mode of practice to teach a procedure is an appropriate approach in each given context.

The importance and complexity of educational judgement in teaching

Educational judgements are at the heart of wise educational practice. They will be called for both in the planning and the execution stage of teaching. Mostly, however, they are invisible and tacit, because when they are sound, appropriate and successful, no one watching is even aware they were made. But in order to critique, refine and develop them, it is sometimes necessary to make them explicit. And the good teacher will always be on the alert to use such judgement in the practice setting to shape and direct or to diverge from and explore the original plan at any stage, whenever what emerges as 'educationally required' needs to take precedence.

Indeed, the teacher as juggler in the teaching session has almost simultaneously to debate and decide how to respond to comments, actions and events. This is a version of reflection-in-action (see Schön 1987). Here, the teacher is constantly torn between competing and incompatible pedagogical demands. For example, the teacher's autonomy is important (teachers should not be the operators of others' policies), but yet there are always compromises to be made and pressures to bend to — even if only temporarily. Indeed, the autonomy intrinsic to teaching is achieved through a balance of its multiple competing and conflicting obligations, not in spite of them or by coming to an inflexible decision to ignore them. Yet if the freedom to teach is also the freedom to withhold teaching from anyone or any group, then how can the task of teaching be both responsible and free?

In the teaching event, there is much to keep re-balancing. For example, the needs of one learner may jeopardize the needs of another. In orchestrating a teaching session there are always competing educational purposes and methods to work around. Teachers must think on their feet, and how successful they are will be determined by the quality of their educational judgements. For example in working with even one learner, let alone several at the same time, there are decisions to be made in how to respond to them. Here the teacher has to:

▷ adapt plans to come closer to what the learner now needs

▷ switch strategies and approaches

▷ keep an eye on the longer-term results of what is happening now

▷ balance freedom and order; behaving like a major authority or setting a nurturing security

▷ sense how far to let one idea run at the expense of another (balancing depth and breadth)

▷ decide whether to go for broad coverage or detail on a smaller scale

▷ decide whether to improvise or go for the pre-set agenda

▷ follow the plan or pursue one learner's questions (especially if there are others not interested in that question)

▷ balance continuity of an argument begun with accepting other colleagues' or learners' comments or questions

▷ balance the teacher's authority with the learner taking the initiative

▷ balance monologue with dialogue

▷ balance group learning with individual learning (attend to the needs of one group member or of all)

▷ decide from whom to reduce attention in order to give it to others (which others, and why?)

▷ decide what a learner is actually asking

▷ know whether learning has taken place and how educationally worthwhile it was.

The most difficult of all these matters is that there are always costs and benefits to every choice a teacher makes. Sometimes the making of such fine judgements 'on the spot' is helped if one has met the issue beforehand either in practice or in one's own thinking. This is but one of many reasons to have thought through one's own personal educational philosophy.

Reflecting on and evaluating the teaching/learning process

The kinds of reflective and evaluative questions that teachers ask themselves about their work, during, as well as after the teaching event, are influenced by their educational understanding, and inevitably will shape what they learn from that work. Thus those working in the technical mode of practice will concentrate upon their skills, techniques and strategies, whilst those working in the moral mode of practice will recognize two important starting points that lay the foundation for the quality of the reflection on teaching/learning events. The first is about whether the event (for both learners and teachers) was *educationally worthwhile*. The second relates to the educational quality of the aims and intentions. Of these two, technically-oriented teachers will be unaware of the first and will not focus for long, if at all, on the second. Both of these areas generate and are linked to questions, as follows, and both are the means of ensuring the educational quality of the whole experience. A single learner is exemplified in the list below, but in the case of more than one, each learner's need would have to be considered.

▷ In what way did the event / activity / session *seek* to provide an educationally worthwhile opportunity for the learner and the teacher?

▷ To what extent did it achieve this and what was educationally worthwhile about it for the learner and the teacher (compared, say to a basic training event)?

▷ Were sound educational aims and intentions set beforehand, were they related to the learner's curriculum and the learner's starting points, and were they shared with the learner?

▷ Was the teaching focus/content appropriate for: that learner and their development; that learner's curriculum; the context of the current placement; and the patients within it?

▷ How were the learner's starting points for this event ascertained?

▷ Was the learner's oral engagement appropriately thoughtful and positive, and why?

▷ Were the moral dimensions of education, and of medicine — as well as the technical ones — properly attended to? (Did the session attend to both ontological matters — the 'being' of the doctor, as well as to epistemological matters — the knowledge and skills needed in medicine?)

▷ Was the learning event appropriately seated within a learning process that included: pre-preparation by teacher and directed preparation by the learner; explicit follow-up work for the learner that was appropriately educational; and arrangements for managing both response to the follow up and also the continuity of learning?

▷ Were educationally sound methods for enhancing learning properly employed?

▷ Were appropriate educational resources provided, were they used at an appropriate time for the learner, and how were they educationally useful?

▷ What did the learner's reflective evaluation of the session (both at the time and in retrospect) say about all these matters?

▷ To ensure the continuity of learning for both teacher and learner, were appropriate written records made — by teacher as a result of the teacher's reflections, and by the teacher and the learner together in recording the learner's activities, achievements and recognizing the next steps necessary?

Thinking, of the kind prompted by these questions, is important for the teacher to engage in, as a means of ensuring the quality of teaching and learning, as well as for the development of educational practice. For the teacher, such thinking about the quality of the education being offered will be occurring beforehand, during and after the teaching/learning event. The kinds of questions offered above will sometimes be at the front and sometimes more at the back of the teacher's mind. Not every session will require detailed written notes about this, but from time to time reflections using these questions should be recorded in writing, both for quality assurance processes and for appraisal.

For the sake of continuity and coherence, the PGME teacher also needs to begin to become more aware of the importance of keeping in a file some brief and informal written and dated record of both their own planning and also the learner's weekly journey (their achievements, on-going progress and next steps to be taken). This is not generally seen as significant where teachers are involved in what I have called 'edu-action' and learning is seen as a random activity to be engaged in pragmatically, when the learner is available. For quality teaching as offered by the advanced teacher however, such record keeping is more significant. Here, again the advanced teacher will need to begin to act as their own agent in this, since keeping such records is not, currently, a requirement.

These matters of course, are also grist to the mill of establishing and keeping updated one's own personal educational philosophy.

Developing your own educational philosophy

We know that education is a values-based enterprise and that our personal and professional values are what drive all our pedagogic decisions. Indeed, our educational values shape how we conduct ourselves as a teacher in the clinical setting. It is thus important, in constructing (and keeping under review) one's educational philosophy, to take careful account of such values especially in respect of what, for us, counts as enduringly worthwhile and important. Complex though values are, they are central and *fundamental to the nature of professional practice and its expertise*. We therefore should begin any attempt to understand and develop our educational philosophy, by exploring them. This can be done by looking first at the visible elements of what we do as a teacher, and then at the more tacit ones. We should also remember that what we *do* says more about what we believe is important than what we *say*, and that colleagues and learners can read this well.

Sometimes our *actions* as teachers reveal educational values that are different from those we would *say* we hold. Here there is a gap between our espoused values (values we claim to hold) and our values-in-use (values that emerge from our practice). In fact it is rare to find that our espoused educational values and our educational values-in-use are totally in harmony but it is something to strive for. When we recognize such a values gap, it is always worth exploring further both our practice and our values.

The following questions — as well as those in the section above — are worth considering while seeking to express a personal educational philosophy.

▷ What do I value as central to good teaching in the clinical setting?

▷ What do I believe about medical practice and the education for it?

▷ What have I learnt about myself as a teacher of PGME?

▷ What are my strengths as someone who fosters the learning of practising doctors?

▷ What do I value as a working clinician? How do I highlight this in my teaching?

▷ What is my vision of how PGME should be practised?

▷ What aspects of practice am I aware of now which I previously took for granted?

▷ What key things about my practice will I now seek to develop?

▷ What key aspects of education have I come to understand better?

▶ What do I now need to work on further in respect of becoming an expert in educational *praxis*?

Chapter ten will now take up some issues associated with reflection and the role of language in learning.

Chapter Ten

Enriched learning in medical practice: nurturing the learner as a person and a clinician

> To guarantee a two-way conversation occurs and to ensure productivity of the teaching session, it is particularly important not to neglect the first stage of the educational process: preparation. With considered and explicit pre-session tasks, the learner can arrive with a common language and a knowledge base which the teaching session can look to develop and expand. This is also a means to understanding the learner better.
>
> Another PG Cert course member

Introduction
Studying the learner
The role of language in learning
Principles for engaging learners in educational dialogue
Some principles for improving learning
Reflection as a central means of learning in and through service

Introduction

This chapter picks up and considers the four main principles for engaging in educationally worthwhile teaching and learning that were listed but not attended to in chapter nine (see p. 142). Given that studying the learner was one such important principle, a range of ways of seeing and understanding the learner is here offered with an indication of what learner-centred teaching actually means (as opposed to how it is sometimes seen in PGME). Since two of the principles that remain to be discussed highlighted the importance of language as the vehicle for learning, this chapter then focuses on the role of language in learning and offers examples of how the raised quality of the teacher's language can promote improved thinking in the learner. Some principles for improving the quality of learning are then presented. Finally, and perhaps most importantly, the chapter focuses on fostering the learner's reflection on themselves as doctors and on their service experiences. Here, reflection is seen as the central means of making meaning from their practice.

Studying the learner

Educationally worthwhile teaching is, by definition, based essentially on sound educational relationships between teacher and learner. This is particularly so in PGME, when working in the moral mode of practice with postgraduates and where the teacher's responsibilities include the development and growth of the learner as a person, and their conduct and moral sensibility as a doctor. Such educational relationships must build the essential basis of mutual respect for each person's rights and dignity and establish the co-operation that enables both parties to explore personal issues like values and professionalism and to establish a safe base from which to face and discuss openly both positive and negative aspects of practice. But what does a 'sound educational relationship' mean here, and how can it be developed?

It means that the educational relationship between learner and teacher is as privileged as that between doctor and patient. It means that between the teacher and their learner is a kind of 'holy ground' that should not be violated by anyone or anything coming between them, by accident or design, to disrupt that special and trusting relationship.

At the heart of a sound and trusting educational relationship is the drive to enable the learner to discover the fullest potential in themselves and to become independent from the teacher. It is certainly not about a dependent relationship where the learner imitates or seeks to become like the teacher. It involves the mutual *working together* of a wise teacher collaboratively with a learner. It requires a learner who is willing not merely to meet the teacher, but where appropriate, to reveal to the teacher the particularity of their understanding and the individuality of their being. This depends more on how the teacher meets the learner, than on the character of the learner. This requires a personal commitment by the teacher that cannot be captured solely in the current language of the 'learning contract'. It is a relationship that goes beyond 'codes of conduct' or guarantees of trustworthiness as safeguarded by professional codes of ethics. At the heart of being a wise teacher are both the motivations and the ethical principles which that teacher brings as a professional educator to the role of 'serving' the learner and fostering their human flourishing.

Such a relationship is developed by a number of means. This includes the ability of the teacher, in order to study the learner, to pick their way through a number of educational complexities and ambiguities and to lose the focus on themselves. Such an approach to education involves the teacher in a commitment to each learner, which (though not limitless) certainly involves active concern, a will to work with rather than on the learner, and a kind of open-ended helpfulness or 'intelligent kindness' (Ballatt and Campling 2011). But it is also about maintaining a respectful distance! This is not about developing dependence by learner on teacher but quite the opposite. The ultimate aim is for the learner to discover themselves more fully and to take on their own learning. This requires balancing a commitment to each learner, with responsibility to all other learners, and (in medical education) to the best interests of patients. As Hansen says: 'In an always delicate and unpredictable way, a teacher needs both closeness to and distance from students in order to serve as a teacher' (Hansen 2001:155-56). He quotes Simon Schama (1996: 96) as saying 'a dispassionate eye is the condition of compassionate intelligence', and goes on to say:

> As a teacher listens to students, reads their work, solves problems with them, and leads them in discussion, he or she learns that students think in distinctive ways about the issues, problems, and possibilities in a subject. Ideally, students are themselves becoming mindful of the very same fact.

> Consequently, teacher and students are, in a manner of speaking, moving closer to one another because they are learning about one another's ways of thinking and acting. But they move closer and closer 'apart', in a crucial moral and intellectual sense, precisely because they discern each other's distinctiveness and individuality. And yet, at the same time, they move farther and farther 'together' into a subject, into a realm of questions, ideas, issues, ways of reading, speaking, seeing, writing, thinking, feeling, and more.
>
> Teachers also move closer and closer apart, and further and further together, as members of a shared practice....
>
> *(Hansen 2001: 156)*

This certainly means a kind of mindful alertness on the part of the teacher. It also means using informal assessment to discover where the learner starts from and therefore where the teacher should begin in tackling a new learning challenge (see below, chapter eleven).

However difficult it might be for the clinical supervisor to establish a sound relationship with their 'trainee' (because of the exigencies of current working procedures in clinical practice) it is an essential basis for quality PGME and should be a priority. Certainly it will bring both teacher and learner huge educational rewards and greater enjoyment in the educational endeavour, and above all conduce to using educational time more profitably. It should also be noted that this way of conceptualizing the teacher/learner relationship is a long way from how 'learner-centred' education is sometimes construed in PGME, where it is erroneously believed that the whole educational enterprise should be shaped by 'what the learner wants'. This idea betrays a lack of awareness of the important distinction between the learner's wants and their needs and even of the ambiguity of the word 'needs'. Indeed failure to recognize this is one of the key characteristics of an unsuccessful teacher.

The learner's needs and interests

As Wilson (1971) long since argued, basing teaching on what the learner says they want is to ignore the blatant fact that in educational terms, knowing what they would like to do, is not the same as knowing what is worthwhile for their education. Thus, even where a learner can declare some 'needs', the teacher will be responsible for selecting from these what is properly appropriate. See also Wilson's critique of Maslow's hierarchy of needs, and his debunking of the idea that the satisfaction of needs is conditional upon the mastering of learning tasks (training and conditioning). He shows that such an approach is both unjustified and highly questionable educationally and that we should not assume that there is nothing unambiguously 'good' about 'meeting children's needs', (Wilson 1971: 11-15).

Wilson's argument is that all 'needs-based education' is compensatory rather than of intrinsic value because it starts by diagnosing what learners 'have not got', and then making up for the deficit. He argues (in critique of behaviourism) that 'the *educative* task of teachers is not to give [learners] a series of shocks followed by motivational pushes and pulls in directions alien to their own, but to try to help them see the significance of goals which already they find interesting and take to be of some possible value' (ibid: 35). Wilson may here be talking about schooling, while PGME is about educating adults, but nevertheless his words are a sharp reminder not to become embroiled in fulfilling the 'needs' of learners as posited by them or others, but to attend rather to learners' interests and to encourage them to be interested in what is intrinsically motivating. Here, of course, as in all else, the teacher is a powerful model.

Clearly, the understanding accrued between teacher and learner during the processes just described, requires rich conversational interaction. In short such understanding can only derive from teacher and learner talking together. This is why the four modes of language (talking and listening as well as reading and writing), have long been acknowledged by professional teachers as quite simply central to the processes of teaching and learning, and as deserving considerable attention in all educational enterprises. As we shall now see, the understanding that arises from language studies in education, which are the *lingua franca* of the professional teacher, is very different and very much more useful than either the tips on questioning found in many medical education text books or the purely technical 'practical' information offered by 'communication skills courses'.

The role of language in learning

Language is both deeply affected by and deeply affects learning. The field of language in education, which studies how language is used in education, has much to offer the advanced teacher in understanding this and using it to educational ends. See writers like Alexander, Barnes, Mercer, Wells and (referenced below, p. 165), backed, of course by the vast field of philosophical work on language in the work of authors like, Bakhtin, Bourdieu, Habermas, Heidegger and Wittgenstein. Also not to be overlooked are writers interested in discourse, like Cameron (2001) and MacLure (2003).

Encouragingly, what might be called a seismic change is coming about in respect of PGME in the 21st century in relation to the role of language in teaching and learning, and this is promoting new educational processes and opportunities. Where teaching postgraduate doctors once rested considerably on the presentational monologue from the teacher, it now increasingly requires a dialogue between teacher and learner — for, as we shall see — a wide variety of educational purposes, including assessment. And as part of this process the learner is beginning to do more of the talking, and becoming more active and interactive. For this to be successful, the teacher needs to become better both at recognizing and utilizing the range of educational resources available, and at listening more carefully to what the learner says.

Resource-based learning and the learner's language

The clinical setting and its broader context (usually the Trust or GP Practice, but perhaps also in future various ambulatory settings) are, of course, the most central and rich resource for PGME. But the *range* of resources this offers and the *range* of learning that could be promoted are often not well recognized (see chapter one above). We showed in Fish and de Cossart (2007), how PGME can become more consciously resource-based, and the learner can be more active in working with the teacher, and that talking is the main vehicle for exploration when teacher is present, while writing and reading are the activities the learner needs to engage in alone, in preparation for and follow up to the discussion with the teacher. This will make for a very different form of conversation with the consultant, and will involve the learner in various kinds of talking and writing. Indeed, the spoken interaction between teacher and learner should lead to further exploration in writing by the learner. This writing (which in most cases will be brief) while primarily for the learner, will also aid both teacher and learner to see what has been made of the resources, ideas and language offered, and will in some cases form the basis of evidence for the learner's portfolio (see chapter eleven).

Resource-based learning is best served by a sequence of activities, which involve the clinical supervisor and a single learner or a small group of two or three learners. Typically, as we suggested in Fish and de Cossart (2007:49-50), these stages are as follows. (The details in this list, because they have been extracted from a deeper discussion, have been made more explicit than in the original text. They are addressed mainly to the clinical supervisor, and with day-to-day practice in mind.)

1. Spot an appropriate learning opportunity which will often be some action or activity of the learner's, observed in the clinical setting and recognized as part of a pattern of conduct already noted as needing educational attention in some way. This will provide the starting point for an important educational conversation.

2. Hold a very brief meeting to highlight the action / activity and agree how learner(s) should prepare for the discussion about it.

3. Offer some sort of resource to guide or encourage the private preparation by the learner(s) for the meeting. This should not be offered judgementally but in the spirit of fuelling a useful two-way discussion. (This may be something brief to read, or something that guides the learner to make bullet points to bring to a discussion in several day's time. See Fish and de Cossart 2007 for plenty of examples, then collect your own.)

4. Engage in that discussion (conversation), the educational aim of which is to ensure *the development of learners' ideas*, which will encourage a change in conduct (not a quick-fix change in behaviour that the learner does not own).

5. Ask for a brief written follow-up on this topic by the learner (which can be emailed to you).

6. Review this with the learner as the record of what has been learnt from this event (by e-mail if not in person).

This enterprise might also from time to time, be added to by the educational supervisor contributing a seventh stage to the process by reviewing the learner's development. This will involve exploring with the learner a summary of key learning points across a given period, for which the learner's portfolio provides more detailed evidence (see chapter twelve below).

If 'resource-based learning', is the centre of this approach to education, interaction with learners in a detailed professional conversation needs to be adopted as a key vehicle for education and the teacher needs to be an expert in a range of language strategies that promote deeper thinking in that learner. This means developing expertise in using language to promote thinking based on an understanding of some important principles. It also means that the teacher will need to guide and support learners to engage in reflection on their own professional and clinical experiences so as to make clinically sound meaning out of them. (This is attended to in the final section of this chapter.)

Talking for learning: some important principles

When the teacher tells a learner, this does not ensure that the learner knows (see for example: Wells 2009; Freire 1970). By contrast, when the learner voices their thinking aloud, the teacher can explore what the learner really understands. To this end, the teacher can initiate at least three types of talk with the learner, as follows.

The presentation or exposition that used to be the vehicle for the teacher to demonstrate their knowledge to the learner, can be used by the learner, while teacher listens carefully and checks out the learner's depth of understanding. But it does require of the teacher careful listening attention and instant diagnosis of the learner's abilities and accuracy. It is about listening and responding by the teacher, not about half listening and at the same time thinking about the important things you are going to say next! Rather the teacher should make brief notes while listening and then pick up the points at the end. Further, this is not something to undertake in the busy clinical setting where the teacher's attention is mainly on something else!

The question and answer session used to be the quick means of checking the learner's knowledge — especially in preparation for the exam. But it was a flawed process. Because the choice of the questions, their order and wording were the teacher's, the learner could second guess answers. Because the speed of the process was usually fast, this precluded an in-depth discussion. And most significantly, the process may have checked aspects of the learner's knowledge but could leave unattended their understanding. Further, today, there are many other means of preparing for exams and the time with a consultant is too valuable to use it for this. This kind of question and answer session might be best used now in the daily clinical supervision and fast instrumentalist interaction, between teacher and learner (see above, p. 140). However, something more educationally worthwhile is more likely to occur by reversing the process, and turning the learner into the questioner.

Discussion in an educationally directed session is the centre of education in PGME. It is usually conducted close to the clinical setting, and only takes place profitably *within it* where that context is an essential resource for the educational interaction. This activity is also referred to as a professional conversation or a dialogue. Dialogue is about enabling the learner to locate him/herself within the unending conversations of culture, community and history. With dialogue comes identity (see Alexander 2004). That is, by talking with another we find ourselves. This fulfils several important learning goals including, as we said above, helping the learner become themselves, getting to know them better and jointly discovering where they are on the pathway of their programme. Its most important role, however, is when the teacher enables the learner to explore and extend their thinking processes about clinical and all other aspects of their work as a doctor. This therefore needs to be privileged in time and space (given a proper amount of time, formally set aside for it, and in an environment which supports serious concentration and deep thinking). And, given its vital role in improving patient safety and care, it needs to happen on a regular basis. Ironically, however, this is the kind of talk that is most frequently neglected, particularly in the current context of healthcare where learners are spending fewer hours with their teachers!

Talking educationally with the learner is thus the meat of education. But such talking can readily veer away from its educational path, can be hijacked by a learner (consciously or unconsciously) in order to avoid an educational challenge or exchange, and can appear to be more educational than it actually is. We should therefore ask ourselves as teachers whether we do provide and promote the right kind of talk to develop the learner. Indeed, we actually have the moral responsibility to find ways of strengthening the power of talk to help our learners think and learn even more effectively than they do.

Since the demands of all this on the teacher are considerable, and the expertise required of them has not been well recognized, the following demonstrates what is needed here.

Principles for engaging learners in educational dialogue

The ideas offered in the following sections have been gleaned and adapted for PGME particularly from the work of Alexander (2004); Barnes (1995); Mercer (1995; 2000); Wells (1999). These ideas and principles can be used for planning purposes, as a prompt for the teacher in a session (perhaps especially one that is grinding to a halt orally), and also to explore one's teaching afterwards by means of investigating what happened via a recording of an educational session. This can be a huge learning activity.

Dialogic teaching comes from the view that knowledge and understanding come from testing evidence, analyzing ideas, and exploring values, rather than unquestioningly accepting somebody else's certainties. It sees the educational interaction with learners as:

▷ *purposeful*: because teachers plan and facilitate dialogic teaching with particular educational aims and intentions in view

▷ *collective*: because teachers and learners address learning tasks together

▷ *reciprocal*: because teachers and learners listen to each other, share ideas, consider alternatives

▷ *supportive*: because teachers and learners need the support of each other to articulate their ideas precisely, freely, and without fear of embarrassment over wrong answers

▷ *cumulative*: because teachers and learners build on their own and each other's ideas and 'chain' them into coherent lines of thinking and enquiry.

Some approaches to building new understanding on past activities, as follows, can be utilized by teachers or learners, as appropriate.

▷ *Consideration of the nuance of the language being used* is an important means of sharpening and refocusing understanding. (For example, how does the term 'delivering care in packages' make us see patients?)

▷ *Recapitulation* is a means of summarizing and reviewing what has gone before. It is at its most educationally powerful when offered by the learner and attended to carefully by the teacher.

▷ *Elicitation* asks a question to stimulate recall and if used collaboratively, rather than as an interrogation, can draw teacher and learner closer together in addressing a problem or an issue of contention.

▷ *Repetition* of the answer from either a teacher or a learner can either give it prominence or may encourage an alternative way of thinking.

▷ *Reformulation* or paraphrasing a learner's response or a teacher's statement can make it more accessible to the other person and encourages improvement of self-expression.

▷ *Reflection, discussion and argument about the answer* can be used to take thinking further.

Using talk educationally, as a means of promoting and developing *thinking*, rather than as a means of 'presenting thinking' that has already happened, is an essential principle for dialogic teaching. This is where the clinical setting is a rich resource in itself, because using what the learner 'has to do' as the basis for discussion will engage them in talking about their thinking. Advice on ways of prompting learners to think more deeply include the following principles.

▷ In planning for teaching it is important to attend to sequence, time and pace in relation to *your* time with learners to get the most out of oral interaction with them.

▷ A collaborative approach to teaching will help the learner to talk something through. This is about seeing as much of one's teaching as possible as a joint enquiry and will open up a dialogue naturally.

▷ The learner, (as well as the teacher), needs to understand that talking is the main means of developing their thinking and reasoning, and that questions that elicit their reasoning and speculation are important and need attending to in detail in order to learn (not in order to show what they already know).

▷ The teacher's role is always to press the learner a little harder, to probe the response, to wait and not to do the thinking for the learner.

▷ It is important to ask the learner 'authentic questions' (those for which the teacher has not pre-specified the answer).

▷ Questions should be worded in order to promote discussion; to clarify or to tackle problems in understanding; to summarize what has been learnt before you move on; to encourage the prediction of what will follow.

▷ There is an important difference between 'interactive pace' and 'cognitive pace'. We all need time to think. Learners need to be disabused of the idea that coming up with a quick answer (irrespective of its quality) will impress the teacher. It is important to recognize the value of stopping and thinking, rather than rushing in.

▷ The teacher's listening skills need to be very good. An educator who listens carefully, recognizes and attends to the learner's agenda first and their own only afterwards.

▷ The tone of voice and register (vocabulary and differing styles of speaking for different audiences) in which the discussion occurs is important. The teacher needs to choose appropriately for different occasions. This means thinking about when an informal conversational style of talk is appropriate, and when something more precise and formal is necessary.

Thus, educational interaction attends to: framing a well-conceived question, giving the learner ample 'wait time' to answer it, and engaging with the answer and responding to it. The following principles should be borne in mind by the teacher. It is important to:

▷ set an atmosphere in which learners can articulate their ideas without fear of embarrassment

▷ give informative diagnostic feedback on which the learner can then build, rather than just saying 'yes' or ;'no' or simply repeating the answer

▷ use reformulation to indicate clearly the *quality* of the answer

▷ use praise discriminatingly

▷ keep lines of enquiry open rather than closing them down.

Where a group of learners engage in discussion in order to understand something new, the following questions in *Frame 10.1 Using talk for collective thinking* are worth considering. It should not be overlooked that this might be useful in a Morbidity and Mortality meeting or any other clinical group discussion related to patient care!

Frame 10.1 Using talk for collective thinking

Choose from the following those questions that are helpful in improving the collaborative thinking of a group. Or set a learning doctor to use them to explore the thinking processes in a particular meeting!

What were your starting points? How did you establish them?

What shared knowledge did you start from?

What was the pattern of your co-operation?

Did you build on the contributions of others?

What were the ground rules for your discussion?

Did you use 'tag' questions ('don't you think?'; 'what do you think?;' 'doesn't it?')

Was talk exploratory?
      Did speakers engage critically but constructively with each other's ideas?
      Was all relevant information offered for joint consideration?
      Where proposals were challenged, were reasons given for alternative views?
      Was agreement sought as the basis for joint progress?
      Was the knowledge made publicly accountable?
      Was the reasoning used made visible in the talk?

Which of the following were characteristic of the discussion:

Mutual exploration	**Explanation**	**Interpretation**
Negotiation	**Enabling**	**Request for help**
Recap	**Eliciting information**	**Overt agreement**
Justifying	**Summarizing**	**Reasoning**
Evaluation	**Resolution**	**New formulations**
Recasting understanding		

Summarizing and meaning-making

Summarizing, giving a concise account of the key points made in a monologue or a conversation, is often used at the end of an interaction but can also be used profitably in the middle. Doctors are assumed to be good at this process because they use it extensively in clinical practice, though several small-scale unpublished investigations by candidates within several PGME Masters Pathways I have taught have raised serious questions about how well this is done! Further, since medicine is an interpretive practice (see Fish 2010; Montgomery 2006), giving a clinical account that is purely factual is impossible. Elements of interpretation will creep in. The teacher who listens to a learner's summary should watch out for this, not to be punitive about it, but to discuss it.

Where the *learner* offers such a summary, in a supportive and nurturing environment, as part of the learning process, this gives the listening teacher a chance to check that they have understood. It also gives the speaker a chance to clarify what has been heard, ensures that the listener takes an active part in what is going on, helps to relate new ideas to ones already held and encourages the critique of both. It will also motivate the learner to listen well during a session, and to consider making brief notes. A learner who knows that they are going to be asked to summarize will listen more carefully. They can then be sure to come away from a conversation with a certain amount of information checked out or a better grasp of ideas that were complex when first heard.

Some principles for improving learning

Much of what teachers need to do to help improve learning is associated with the quality of the language of both teachers and learners in their educational interactions. As Wells (1992) has shown us, learners need to be active in formulating their own questions and developing their own strategies for learning. The following are important principles.

- ▷ Learning is a social and collaborative enterprise.

- ▷ Knowledge is not a commodity, existing in some pure and abstract form in a world independent of learners. It is a state of understanding achieved through constructive mental activity of each individual — in which that individual engages with the ideas they meet.

- ▷ Knowledge never enters the learner's mind in the form in which it was transmitted.

- ▷ Instead, learners progressively construct their own knowledge by bringing what they already know to bear on new information in order to assimilate or accommodate to the new and extend or modify initial understanding.

▷ This process results in (provides each individual with) a personal resource, but its construction is essentially social and cultural.

▷ It is through participation with more mature members of a community in socially (and professionally) significant purposeful activities that learners encounter the knowledge and skills that are valued in their culture and their profession.

▷ This happens via *language* and *activities*.

▷ By learning through co-constructing the meaning of what they have been offered educationally, with their teacher and each other, learners take over the resources and make them their own.

▷ This process of 'appropriation' involves the active transformation of the information provided by 'teacher' and other participants in the activity, and means that the learner's resulting knowledge (or understanding) is never a copy of what was initially offered, but rather a personal reconstruction of it.

▷ As a result the understanding gained may go beyond the initial 'model' offered and learners may find or create new meanings and solutions to problems and even formulate new problems.

Thus education is mediated through language (talking, listening, reading and writing). It requires a purposeful linguistic interaction with others such that meaning-making occurs for the learner and the teacher. This also injects interest and energy into a teaching interaction because it allows for unexpected and unpremeditated outcomes for both teacher and learner, in sharp contrast to the boring drudgery of a product view of teaching (see above, p. 149) where all is predictable. However, we should also remember that commonality of (shared) reference is not automatically assured by all this, because learners' different backgrounds, cultural and life experiences, concerns and interests, will ensure that participants in shared interaction will nonetheless always speak with different voices, and this difference should be valued by the teacher. It does mean, however, that we all have to work to achieve and maintain a shared *intersubjective* understanding of the matter in hand. This requires us to be able to see as the other person sees.

Reflection as a central means of learning in and through service

Reflection has long been recognized as a central means of learning from experience or practice. It requires an exploratory cast of mind, which is critical, rigorous and meticulous. It is about:

▷ seeking to uncover rigorously and understand and articulate the *relationship* between one's visions, values and beliefs, and one's thought, knowledge and action, in reference to specific examples of one's own practice

▷ having an exploratory cast of mind, that is both critical and meticulous

▷ processes which crucially include: contextualising one's practice; viewing and investigating it critically; and exploring open-mindedly how it relates to wider understandings of that practice and the practice of one's profession.

▷ understanding our practice better, and thus being motivated and committed to improving it, and thereby being equipped to go about such improvement.

It engages the learner in processes, which can be used as a guide to thinking about an aspect of clinical practice and which crucially includes the following:

▷ contextualizing the practice event carefully and noting the influence of the context on our thinking within that event

▷ viewing and investigating the event critically from a number of perspectives

▷ exploring open-mindedly how that which is learnt from the event also relates to wider understandings of our own practice and the practice of our profession

▷ coming to understand our practice better, and thus being motivated and committed to improving it, and being equipped to go about such improvement.
(See Fish and de Cossart 2007).

Reflective practice is a special kind of practice, which involves systematic critical enquiry into one's professional work and one's relationship to it. Put another way it is about engaging in an emancipatory educational experience (de Cossart and Fish 2012). This approach to practice is also related to the Aristotelian term *praxis*, which is about morally informed action, or action shaped by critical consideration of both its ends and means. This involves standing back from that practice (and ourselves as part of that practice) and viewing as an observer might, both the practice and our beliefs, assumptions, expectations, feelings, attitudes and values as they impact on our practice.

Reflection enables learners (in respect of specific *selected events* of practice) to:

▷ explore, make sense of, and thus understand more fully their experience, actions and events

▷ contextualise this current experience and relate it critically to other relevant theory and practice

▷ extend their current competence in clinical practice

- recognize new challenges to work on, in clinical practice

- appreciate the subtleties of clinical practice (eg: the gap between espoused values and values-in-use)

- connect particular practice experiences, events and activities to wider ideas and ideals of practice across their profession

- develop a personal vision of clinical practice

- provide evidence of growing insight and progress in understanding

- crystallize and summarize progress at the end of various stages of learning.

None of this is about a 'cosy' unstructured chat over tea, but involves a rigorous investigation that explores systematically all aspects of a piece of practice, in order to understand it better (unlike audit, which investigates an event to pinpoint and deal with problems).

Some defining characteristics of reflective practice

The key characteristics of good and successful reflection on practice, in all contexts within professional practice, are as follows.

- The subject matter should be one's own practice and its particular context.

- Reflection may be on everyday events, or on the conditions that shape action and thought.

- Reflection may focus on an on-going experience or a 'one-off' event.

- It is likely to be triggered by uncertainty about something in the mind of the practitioner.

- It will engage with moral and ethical content (professional work being morally centred).

- It will be precipitated by questions / tasks / personal considerations / problematic issues, to which there is no *simple* solution.

- It will have strongly critical elements.

- Its end point is the attainment of better understanding in the context of improving practice generally.

- It is not just about thinking, but articulating that thinking in spoken or written form and as a result being able to extend, refine and develop it.

▷ It is enhanced when shared with others.

These are the general matters about reflection that are the case irrespective of the context in which reflection occurs or the kind of practitioner involved. Fish and de Cossart have produced details of reflection especially tailored to the needs of doctors, which they refer to as 'clinical reflection'. A detailed approach to clinical reflection for doctors will shortly be offered in three separate publications for three different audiences: undergraduate doctors; postgraduate doctors with no previous experience of using reflection for PGME purposes; and postgraduate doctors who are familiar with the processes of using The Invisibles (see Fish and de Cossart 2007) and Clinical Reflective Writing (see: www.ED4MEDPRAC.co.uk).

There is a debate to be had about the role of the Arts in supporting reflection on practice by postgraduate doctors. For a useful discussion of this see Downie (1999) and Evans (2001).

The following chapter now takes up the enterprise of illustrating the thinking that informs wise educational practice and which advanced teachers should engage in. It provides practical examples of the outcomes of this, in respect of informal assessment.

Chapter Eleven

Enriched *informal* assessment: diagnosing where learners are, thus enabling more focused teaching

I recently asked hospital consultants on a PG Cert course to reconstruct a set of ideas that we had discussed together in detail in the previous teaching session. They were given the outline of a diagram to help them, but none of the detail. When we explored their completed attempts at this, the group went through a series of interesting emotions.

Firstly, they faced the fact that they had struggled to reconstruct the details and none had been totally successful. Then they complained that if only they had been told the night before that they were 'going to be tested', they would have learnt it by rote and been almost totally successful in their work! Clearly, they perceived all such exercises as a serious test — a memory test — *where success in the set task* (no matter its educational value) mattered most of all. They even saw it as a possible attempt to 'catch them out'.

It took them some time to see that the point of the exercise had been for us both (learners and teacher) to see just where they were in the complex journey from meeting a new idea in the first place, through having a grasp of some of it, followed by developing their own overall knowledge of it in their own words and then on to understanding it so that it related to their other ideas and they could re-create it for someone else. In this journey to understanding, the role of a test that required regurgitation of someone else's words would have been minor indeed, since no such memory test could possibly have clarified the quality of their understanding.

Their response to this was mainly because the concept of *informal assessment* as such (where the point is to establish where the learner is in understanding) was alien to them as not being central to PGME curricula. Yet such assessment is both an indispensible means for each learner to recognize where they are personally in grasping something new, and also an equally indispensible means for the teacher to identify a meeting point from which they can, together, successfully continue their educational journey.

Introduction
Informal and formal assessments and how they relate to formative and summative assessments
Using informal assessment to study the learner and promote learning
Some examples of the design of informal assessments
The quality and use of informal formative assessment
Endnote

Introduction

Chapter eight in Part One provided a basis for *thinking* more deeply about assessment than many senior clinicians usually have time to do. It argued that rather than merely seeing assessment as a means of using 'given' national tools to measure the learner's achievement, thus treating it as separate from learning and teaching, there is need to use it to promote and motivate learning and to provide an important basis for planning the next learning and teaching experiences. This chapter therefore, seeks to consider and illustrate how *informal* assessment might be used to promote and improve the education of learning doctors. That is, it explores informal assessment from an educator's viewpoint, rather than from a more purely technical one. The next and final chapter (chapter 12), considers *formal* assessment from the same viewpoint. This looks at the national assessment requirements within each learner's curriculum, which are part of the learners' entitlement and therefore must be properly attended to. It then shows how, with greater understanding of the principles of assessment, these assessment 'tools' can also be enriched as serious learning opportunities.

Both this chapter and the next see assessment as central, not just as an adjunct, to teaching and learning, and as impoverished when separated from them. Each chapter addresses the question: how, by drawing on their educational understanding, can PGME teachers use assessment *more educationally* to the benefit of learners and learning? Both chapters illustrate how without engaging in a root and branch revolution, current assessment processes can be evolved so as to become more educationally worthwhile.

This chapter, then, argues that teachers not only can and sometimes tacitly do, but actually explicitly should, as part of their moral practice, use informal assessments to promote learning. This can be achieved by creating active opportunities within their day-to-day teaching for individual learners to undertake tasks designed by their individual teacher in order to reveal their immediate learning needs, as highlighted by the particular context in which they work. This kind of learning activity is already common practice in PGME, but is clearly not always understood by either party as a key educational strategy and sometimes (as reported in the box at the front of this chapter), it is misread by learners as designed to catch them out! Using *informal* assessment *educationally* puts learning first and uses assessment as a part of an overall educational process. Such assessments (unlike those required within the national PGME curricula) are the province of and are under the control of individual teachers to construct and use as they see appropriate. But they only achieve their educational goal when the learner understands their purpose.

In exploring these issues, this chapter begins with a careful delineation of the differences between formative and summative assessment and how they relate to formal and informal assessment. Some key principles are then offered, enabling the teacher to introduce the learner to the notion of informal assessments and the design of small educational activities that will assess the learner's current understanding and pave the way for more enriched and appropriate day-to-day teaching.

Embedded in the presentation of these assessment principles is a practical indication of how they may be used to design informal motivating assessments that promote learning. Examples are then given of specific informal assessments, which show how the teacher can easily design their own in order to challenge the learner and extend their learning. The chapter will end with some comments on building quality into educational forms of informal assessment in the clinical setting.

Informal and formal assessments and how they relate to formative and summative assessments

Informal assessments

This section begins with a stark warning. Informal assessment of a learner can be and often is, casually formed on the basis of flimsy evidence and subsequently used in an undisciplined and anti-educational way. This occurs when a teacher allows impressionistic and unchecked interpretations of a learner's abilities, based on a one-off occasion, to cloud their judgements about the learner's overall potential and achievements. Of course, we cannot help forming impressions of colleagues and learners as we meet and work with them, but before we attach any significance to these, we should always seek to test them out for fairness and accuracy against concrete evidence over a period of time, just as clinicians would check out their clinical intuitions in respect of patients.

By contrast to this, informal assessment *used educationally,* is a natural part of good teaching. Such assessment processes provide information about learners' current understanding and help the teacher to reconsider their next plans or to reshape their next educational interactions with the learner. These processes might begin by looking over the learner's shoulder to see what they are writing or (in clinical practice) doing. But this needs to be done diagnostically in respect of learning and the learner, not only in respect of supervising their *clinical* practice. More carefully considered informal assessment activities need to be designed by a teacher so that, in a nurturing setting, the learner can be prompted to discover what they really understand and what they need more help with, and the teacher can understand how to proceed.

This kind of informal assessment activity can only be designed by a specific teacher for a given learner and should be positioned carefully within the planned learning event. Such a process, with its formative purpose, is not suitable to be part of a summative assessment. Thus, informal assessment is actually 'informal formative assessment', and is always 'off the formal record'. This means that the results are not *directly* recorded, though teachers may write about them for their learners' eyes only and they may also (along with many other kinds of evidence) use the results indirectly, to *inform* their judgement when writing the formal report on the learner's achievements during the course of the attachment.

Such informal assessments need to be created by the teacher who engages the learner in interesting activities to complete on their own, that will allow the learner enough opportunity to reveal, in their own way and their own order, the scope of their current understanding. As we saw in chapter ten above, teacher-directed questioning does not achieve this. In fact, informal assessment tasks are already easily available as part of the resources found in any clinical setting. Spotting the potential of these for informal assessment purposes, as they occur, is an important aspect of teaching. But informal assessments can also be invented or created by the teacher, and, since these are likely to be re-useable for other learners in that specialty, they can also be made robust (by, for example, lamination) and stored ready for future use.

Knowing and coming to understand

Informal assessment is a useful means of diagnosing where their learner is, in 'coming to understand' rather than merely being able to regurgitate a range of medical knowledge. This is because 'knowing' and 'understanding' are not one and the same thing, any more than 'knowing' and 'believing', or 'remembering' and 'understanding' are the same. In PGME, many if not most teachers make many un-informed and un-based assumptions about knowledge and knowing and how to acquire these, and don't even know they are making them! Further, 'knowing' itself is a complex concept because it can mean anything from having a mere acquaintance with the look or sound of something, to knowing it intimately and/or broadly. Thus 'coming to know' is also a more complex process than is usually recognized in PGME, where telling someone seems to be seen as sufficient to enable them to know.

The following is a list of misapprehensions about coming to know.

▷ If you tell someone something, then of course, they will know it.

▷ If they don't *then* know it, there is something wrong with them.

▷ You can 'give' someone your knowledge by transferring it to them.

▷ It is best to tell them *now in one session* everything they need to know (all that you know).

▷ They will thus come to know something — or even everything!

▷ This means that they will make a direct leap from 'not knowing' to 'knowing'.

▷ Knowledge is absolute and unchanging, so once they know it, they will be unchallengeably knowledgeable about it.

▷ Knowledge lies in books and in 'knowledgeable' people, so you learn simply by reading and by being told.

▷ Once you know something, you will always know it, as long as you have a good memory.

▷ Knowing something is the same as understanding it and being able to use it.

By contrast to these statements, educators know that 'coming to know something someone else knows' is a complex process. It might begin by being alerted to some new knowledge through reading or listening. Such knowledge could merely be committed through repetition to rote memory. But this gives no evidence of the grasp of even the basic meaning of it, let alone having any real understanding of it, and certainly no evidence of being able to put it into use. Knowledge needs to be studied. This involves trying to understand it for example by talking – by means of putting it into one's own words and checking that these words are a reasonable reconstruction of the original, and also by trying to put the given knowledge into practice. This often initially involves keeping the page open whilst working with the knowledge, and then later referring only to the knowledge 'in one's head', whilst operationalizing it.

Being tested on new knowledge out of the blue, then, by being asked to regurgitate what has been learnt, is of little use in the early stages of meeting new knowledge (although it can alert the learner to just how much more they need to take in about something). Equally, in the later stages of understanding something, it is almost an insult to ask for its simple regurgitation. However, asking for it to be used on the spot in a problem-solving exercise can be very revealing. Equally, asking for a critique of that knowledge and how it relates to other known ideas or practices can also be a useful process in diagnosing the learner's next needs. Thinking about 'knowledge' critically, and learning to distinguish the valuable and trustworthy from the persuasive but glib and unfounded, also takes practice and experience during which the learner may need a teacher's help.

Thus, helping the learner to come to know something (to develop understanding) requires both learner and teacher to engage in a variety of processes that move the learner from merely knowing about something to gaining deep understanding of it and being able to use it and critique it. During this process, it is the learner and not the teacher who needs to do most talking, and, again, the teacher needs to listen very carefully to the learner. This is a complete reversal of the normal power relationships in PGME, and it takes practice for it to become a natural process. Teachers should thus be careful, especially whenever something unexpected happens, not revert to their old 'default' position of 'teller'!

Formal assessment

By comparison to informal assessment, formal assessment is not personalized to a learner to help them in struggling with the process of coming to understand. Rather, it looks at the product of learning. Formal assessment uses methods (referred to in the technical mode of practice as 'tools'), that have been pre-designed outside the teaching context and which are applied to all candidates — sometimes, but not always, at the same time. Its purpose is to gather apparently objective evidence about an individual's and a cohort's achievements, and to place these on record in order to judge them in the light of an agreed (but in reality arbitrary) 'national standard'. Such assessment can occur at set and discrete stages during an educational programme. The methods of formal assessment can be used both formatively (during) and summatively (at the end) of the teaching/learning process. But either way, the results of formal assessment are always 'on the record'.

Formal formative and summative assessment

Formal formative assessment, which uses standard national assessment during learning, is pre-designed for formal purposes in order to gain on-the-record evidence of the learner's ability at points along the learning pathway of the educational programme. Like all informal assessment, it should shape the subsequent teaching and learning and influence the demands to be made in future on that learner. But being pre-designed and therefore general, it picks up only how the individual learner relates to trends predicted by curriculum designers, and is not sensitive to the more detailed contextual needs of the individual learner. By capturing how a learner is progressing during the programme (at about the mid-point of the programme), formal formative assessment also will flag up the need for any remediation necessary for learners who are not making normal progress, in time for that remediation to occur before the end of the programme.

Summative assessment, by comparison, is always a 'final' judgement made at the end of a particular programme or stage of that programme, based on whether — at a given end-point — the work meets the published standard (the given end-goal at a given time), such that the learner has passed or completed satisfactorily that phase of education. (Standards, it should be remembered however, are in fact arbitrary notions!) Although summative assessment is treated as a formal process that creates 'final' formal evidence on the record, such 'final' assessment should never rest on a one-off process — even where it includes a final exam. The learner's end achievements are the result of progress over a period, and are also their starting point for the next stage.

Final assessment should rest upon transparent formal evidential perspectives and these should be collected along the way. Portfolios provide a useful means of presenting this evidence, but they are only robust if they are designed with that purpose in mind. In PGME, summative assessment happens at the end of each attachment and also at the end of each key stage of the curriculum (Foundation, Core and Specialty stages). Until the final completion of all this, the summative assessment from the previous stage *should* become part of the formative evidence for the start of the next stage, (though it seems in practice that it is not always explored in any detail by teachers at that next stage up). More about this will be found in the following chapter.

The inescapable significance of the assessor's judgement

It is vitally important to remember that all assessments rely somewhere along the line on the professional judgement of the teacher/assessor. There is no process that can totally rid assessment of subjectivity and even some form of bias. Education is not a science. Learning is neither a scientific nor an incremental process. An individual's learning does not conform to a pre-charted pathway but happens in fits and starts as they meet personal learning plateaux and unexpected race tracks. Thus the results of assessment are at best temporary and educational judgement is an *inescapable* element of the assessment process, even where scripts are machine-marked (because judgement informs how the technology has been set up).

Further, since all learners are different, the stage they have reached at the key assessment points will not be entirely predictable, nor can it accurately predict later success or failure Thus, no assessment can ever be totally objective and none can be totally accurate. Because of this, 'good assessment practice has to recognize the tentative nature of judgements made about ... achievements', (Murphy 2002: 179). This is why Broadfoot speaks of the 'myth of measurement' (Broadfoot 2002).

Good educational practice holds that whatever other purposes they serve, all assessments should seek to develop the learner's ability to self-assess and provide the teacher with important feedback on the quality of their own as well as the learner's work. This will help them tailor the next teaching they offer more specifically to the learner's immediate needs, but cannot be relied upon in the longer term.

Using informal assessment to study the learner and promote learning

Any system of assessment must be coherent and principled. The selection of such principles is of course also values-based. In the moral mode of educational practice, where the role of assessment is to promote learning, we need to think about assessment first and foremost in terms of what opportunities it offers to students to extend their learning and demonstrate their progress, as well as how that helps teachers understand where they begin so as to shape their next teaching. A number of important key principles follow from this that enable us to re-shape assessment so as to be educational for the learner.

The educational purposes of informal assessment

Defining and agreeing the *purposes* of assessment is a vital starting point in designing that assessment. Discussion between teachers and learners about the general purposes of informal assessment might serve to make more open and transparent any negative views learners might bring to the process, so that they can be addressed. Essentially, informal assessment is purely to help the learner and the teacher to engage together in more focused and better tailored educational interactions. It might also help highlight the merits and the educational point of the interactions between teacher and learner.

The following principles might be a useful guide for teachers designing informal assessments for their learners. They are not difficult either to understand or to use in designing creative activities for the learner. Such activities can occur to any teacher who thinks for a few minutes about how to engage the learner in thinking more deeply about what they have been taught. Indeed, for the advanced teacher, there can be pleasure in the creativity they are called upon to use in designing new activities. The order of the following principles is important.

1. The use of informal assessment needs to be negotiated and agreed by

each teacher with their learner in principle at the start of the educational programme as a natural part of their educational interaction. (This can be part of the learning agreement.)

2. The learner should understand the nature of informal assessment as a teaching/learning strategy whose results are 'off the record'.

3. Its benefits to both the learner and the teacher need to be understood by both (though the learner may have to trust the teacher at the start that these will become clear).

4. Informal assessment needs to have a very clear educational purpose that is understood by teacher and learner.

5. The exact role it will play in any given teaching and learning session needs to be clear in the teacher's and the learner's mind.

6. The timing of the informal assessment within the teaching/learning session, should be considered carefully, in order to maximize both its benefits and the educational time teacher and learner spend together.

7. Informal assessment activities can occur as part of preparation for or follow-up to a teaching interaction with a learner, as well as during the session. This will depend on the above principles and also whether or not the teacher can benefit from being present to observe and listen to the learner during the informal assessment.

8. The teacher needs to review the choices available to someone designing or re-designing assessment *for educational purposes*, and where necessary to understand how to critique or defend their selection.

The choices available are illustrated by asking whether the assessment is:

▷ convergent or divergent: (narrowly focused or requiring creativity of the learner)

▷ summative or formative: (at the end of the learning or integral to it)

▷ quantitative or qualitative: (producing numbers, or using words, diagrams or pictures)

▷ objective or subjective: (some say there is no such thing as objectivity)

▷ written, oral, diagrammatic or some other creative form

▷ requiring a pre-set format, or one that the learner can choose.

The reasons for these choices are also important. For example: sometimes writing is used to show what has already been learnt, *but*, sometimes the learning is *in* (endemic to) the key processes of writing because new understanding comes as we redraft. It should be noted that inviting the learner to choose a medium can provide refreshing new perspectives.

These principles and questions are intended to help the teacher to match the nature of the assessment activity set to the educational purposes agreed between teacher and learner and then to create appropriate details as discussed below.

Informal assessment activities that challenge the learner to use and extend learning

Teachers in PGME have far more control over informal formative assessments than over the formal assessments found in 'Tools of the Trade'. Informal assessment is a process that enables the teacher to take local *educational* control of the curriculum (as opposed to simply conforming to its technical demands).

Informal formative assessment can be designed by the teacher as a natural part of the teaching / learning process and can occur before and throughout the time that teaching and learning is happening. The supportive nature of the *learning context* in which formative assessment takes place is a critical element in engaging the learner in this process. Formative assessment which involves informing the teacher about what sense the learner is making of what they are offered — without making *or recording* any final judgements about this — allows teachers to make decisions and monitor their teaching based on learners' responses. The purpose of formative assessment is to lead to further learning. If it fails in this, then the intention was formative, but the process was not.

The fact that informal assessment is formative and off the record, releases teacher and learner from the tyranny of engaging in assessments that are about 'having to get it right'. It allows teacher to design educational activities that the learner need not regard as crucial to providing formal evidence of their progress, so that they can experiment, take risks, try out ideas and thus discover more about themselves as learners and what they know, understand, can do and achieve.

For the teacher this means the opportunity to see how the learner thinks, to distinguish what the learner actually understands from simply what they know, to see what sense they have made of learning components and whether they have properly seen how to inter-relate them and synthesize them. In short, informal assessment can crucially be used to explore not just what learners know and can do but whether and in what ways they can use what they have learnt. Well designed informal assessments can be fun, can be motivating, can enrich the relationship between teacher and learner (because they enable both to reveal themselves as people), and can provide teacher and learner with deeper insight about how best to proceed next in the educational adventure.

Some examples of the design of informal assessments

Any teacher can design informal assessment processes which are broadly formative in nature, to any chosen educational purpose for any individual learner. It is part of the process of engaging the learner actively. It involves creating activities for the learner to engage in that make visible and provide diagnostic information about the following:

- ▷ the learners' thinking, decision-making processes and judgement

- ▷ the depth of their understanding

- ▷ their use of knowledge and ability to synthesize it in practical situations

- ▷ their ability to be pro-active

- ▷ their ability to think ahead

- ▷ their ability to see the wider picture.

This should be regarded as part of the creative process of planning for facilitating learning, and requires the clinical supervisor to think like an educator (see above, chapter nine). Some of these informal assessments may be oral or on paper, where the evidence can be reviewed and easily used diagnostically. Some however, will be activities that relate to working in the clinical setting. Here the clinical supervisor needs to be thinking both as clinician (ensuring the safety of patients) but also not forgetting to think as an educator, using the clinical event to diagnose the learners' abilities and educational needs.

Getting the learner to draw and talk about a diagram or use a given model to explain something newly learnt

In a range of contexts and for a range of different kinds of knowledge, it can be useful to ask a learner to construct and label a diagram to explain something they have learnt, or to use a given anatomical or other model, to explain something newly learnt. This is best done in front of the teacher at an appropriate time within a teaching session and with the learner talking as they draw or point to the model.

If a learner-generated diagram is a reproduction of something that the learner originally met as a diagram, this would be mere regurgitation or at best show where the learner is in a very new piece of knowledge. It may be better that the learner is asked to create a new diagram in order to elaborate what has been learnt, and to link it to what was known before, and/or also to show the relationship between things that have been newly learnt. The benefits here are that the learner *uses* the knowledge and the teacher can readily see and hear how far the learner understands something. This may need to occur early in a teaching session to direct the next stages or it may fulfil a reviewing or summarizing process near the end of a session.

Thus this process of the learner concocting and explaining a diagram can be convergent or divergent: summative or formative; and in either a teacher- or a learner-chosen format. It thus combines both the written and oral but in a form that is easy to produce 'off the cuff'. Here the only preparation required by the teacher is to make a simple decision about exactly what the task is and how, when and why to present the learner with that task.

Getting the learner to construct a self-assessment grid

In asking the learner to construct a self-assessment grid, the task may be to list what they can and cannot do, or what they can do but do not understand, and rate these in terms of the quality of their skills or knowledge. There are some assessment 'tools' like triggered assessment and the Intercollegiate Surgical Curriculum assessment processes that already set the parameters of such a grid, as the basis for conducting an assessment of a procedure. (See de Cossart and Fish 2005, chapter ten.) Thus this would be used at the start of an assessment session and lead into and act as a base line for the assessment. But a simple version could also be used in preparation for meeting with a supervisor about the learning agreement. So for some educational/ assessment purposes, there would be a set format and for some, the learner might choose the format (and their very choice might be highly informative to the teacher).

Thus this process would usually be in preparation for or at the start of a teaching session. Such an assessment format tends to be technical and convergent, and would normally use figures (bands or percentages). Its educational benefits, beyond the normal diagnostic ones, would include the development of better self-assessment in the learner. Further, like the use of a diagram, it is quickly executed and requires no lengthy writing from the learner or reading from the teacher.

Starting a professional conversation in a novel way rather than following a mantra

The professional conversation, as explored above, is of itself a means of informal assessment, simply because it requires the learner to play a key part in the talking and to contribute also to the content. The benefits of this can be made more striking if the learner is offered a starting point that is different from what is normally used.

For example, instead of starting a conversation about a patient by asking for the normal presentation from the learner, it is possible to start by asking: "what is your professional judgement about the treatment for this patient?" They can then be asked to work backwards to explore their thinking processes that brought them to this point. Alternatively the learner could be asked: "what will you do for the care of this patient?"

Again, because this is a conversation that can be held without preparation and at any point in a teaching session, it is easy to use. It does however require the teacher to listen very carefully not just to the clinical issues, but also to the educational needs of the learner as revealed in their responses. Without this there is a significant danger of agreeing tacitly to something inaccurate offered by the learner.

Using information on cards to prompt the learner to talk and make connections

Here there is need for the teacher to do some preparation, because they need to create a resource to check out the learner's ability in some aspect of their attachment. But once made and laminated, such a resource can be used over and over again by learners as they come to that point of need within their attachment.

Thus the teacher may, for example, choose to make prompt cards or to cut up diagrams or invent cases that are bound to be needed at some point in the normal teaching process. These resources may be in written or diagrammatic form, but the learner can respond orally to them or even 'play' with the relationship between them, and talk about this. Again, of course, the teacher's responsibility is to think diagnostically about the learner's educational needs, rather than treating this as a test or a mere game.

These are merely four generalized examples that the teacher could call upon and by thinking creatively but briefly about them may introduce both a more motivating spirit into the teaching session and be able to learn more about the learner and their educational needs. Put another way, such resources are a key means of enabling the teacher to 'study the learner', which we said in chapter four is an important activity.

The quality and use of informal formative assessment

Both social and cultural factors and teaching / learning factors have a key impact on the quality and use of such informal formative assessment. Some *Social and cultural factors* support formative assessment, and some undermine it as follows.

▷ Learning can be seen as an individual or a collective (group) activity. Where it is a collective activity, formative assessment works well and the learner does not feel exposed. However, learners can hide their individual problems within a crowd.

▷ The way assessment is seen within the national level 'centralized curriculum' affects learners' attitudes to formative assessment. These attitudes need to be discussed openly by teachers and learners. The more controlled the summative assessments are, the less popular can be the formative ones, yet the more useful they are in supporting teaching and learning. Learners may need to be helped to understand this.

▷ Where the main assessments in the curriculum are influenced by performance outcomes or a behavioural objectives approach, formative assessments are of less interest to learners — until they see assessment in a broader light.

▷ The greater the availability of educationally worthwhile resources to promote learning and assessment, the better and more popular are the formative assessments. Teacher needs to develop a collection of these and have them ready to hand in the clinical setting (or nearby).

▷ The culture of the institution and its dominant model of teaching and assessment seriously affects learners' attitudes to formative assessment. Teachers need to discuss assessment at 'faculty' level within a department so that there is a coherent policy that provides learners with a common approach.

▷ Where marks and grades matter more than words, formal summative assessment will be more popular. This is why teachers need to talk to learners about these things and offer them motivating examples of (small) assessment exercises that they enjoy and can see the educational point of. (Offering them this chapter to read and discussing it might be one useful resource to support this.)

The following factors are influential in relating teaching to learning through informal formative assessment.

▷ Informal formative assessment flourishes where there is a supportive but challenging environment and an appropriately open interaction between teacher and learner (where a professional conversation is a tradition).

▷ Anything that militates against learning is a threat to the usefulness of informal formative assessment.

▷ Affective factors are important. Learning involves trust and motivation, requires a safe environment where difficulties can be admitted and constructive responses offered; where there is awareness of the teacher's commitment, and the learner's wish to improve; where there is willingness to be creative and take risks.

▷ Teachers need to be overtly responsive to the achievements that result from a learner's informal formative assessment, because only through this will the process be fully educational and because how one such assessment is handled and responded to by that teacher will affect the learner's attitudes to and success in later assessments of this kind!

▷ Informal formative assessment thrives where there is trust. This is about: trust that the teacher is there to help but will not immediately rescue learner from mistakes or misunderstandings, but where necessary will ultimately offer more enlightenment; and trust that the teacher understands the learner, really knows what is to be learnt, understands the task, and can help the learner to learn.

▷ Informal formative assessment is also about equipping the learner with an understanding of 'where they need to get to' in their learning. It provides the learner with a sense of what to strive for and how that relates to where they currently are.

Good assessment generally rests on getting right the degree of explicitness about what the assessment requires. This demands careful use of words and an awareness of their nuance, and a balance of detail about what the assessments require of the learner. Such detail needs to be not too much, but not too little. It is also important to provide a chance for the learner to *talk* about the requirements of the assessment with teacher before engaging in the task.

Endnote

In this chapter we have explored a principled approach to enriching the practice of teaching, learning and assessment in PGME, through informal formative assessment. This is intended to enable teachers to use assessment in more educational ways. We have also explored practical ways in which teachers can become properly creative about the assessment processes they use to promote learning.

But so far in Part Two, in order to focus sharply on this (and in order to demonstrate some ways of enriching learning and teaching in chapters nine and ten), we have focused on teaching, learning and assessment more-or-less separately, thus teasing apart these three processes whilst at the same time arguing that they are really part of education as a whole. The final chapter will now seek to bring these all together in the context of the formal assessment processes of PGME, and to show how the 'tools of the trade' could be relocated into the moral mode of practice.

Chapter Twelve

Enriched *formal* assessment: using better teaching and learning to enhance the required 'tools'

As a trainee who has used workplace-based assessments (WBPAs) since her Foundation programme, I have witnessed their impact first hand. Unfortunately, from my own experience and through talking to others, these assessments are treated by most as a laborious task that ultimately serves to be a 'boxticking' exercise. ... Indeed, looking back through my teeming portfolio filled with WBPAs I realised that I cannot remember doing some of them.

Whilst I understand that some sort of evidence is required to show the progress of a trainee, one does question the educational benefit of a generic assessment that is marked on a single A4 sheet, filled with boxes waiting to be ticked. ...

From my experience, the importance attached to these assessments appears to be more of a 'Has the trainee performed the requisite number?' ... I have never once been questioned about the quality of the assessments I have undertaken or what I have learned from them.

Dr Kirat Guliani, in Meara and Guiliani (2011): 257

The processes that have enhanced the CBD provide a lot more learning for trainers about the trainee — about where they are.

Consultant Paediatrician

It has changed me, and the way I think about my cases.

New Consultant in Emergency Medicine

Introduction
The formal assessment 'tools' for workplace based assessment (WPBA) in PGME
The Foundation Curriculum (2012) and how it relates to earlier versions
Making these assessment processes more educational
The significance of portfolios: some ideas for the future
Last words

Introduction

This final chapter explores the formal assessment procedures for PGME, in the light of the principles that guide educational assessment as offered in chapters eight and eleven above. The formal assessment requirements for PGME, the ineptly named 'Tools of the Trade', were set down originally by MMC. Although there has been some small development of them, as exemplified by the 2012 Foundation Curriculum, they still attend to the performance of the learner without setting this fully in an educational context and with little emphasis on their educational (as opposed to the administrative) benefits.

This chapter will explore the current contribution of these formal 'assessment tools' to the postgraduate education of doctors. It will demonstrate that it is very possible to enrich them so that both learner and teacher gain something educationally worthwhile from them, and so that what they place on record is more educationally valuable. To this end, it begins with an analysis and critique of the character and philosophy of the 'tools' more generally, and then looks in detail at their latest development, by examining the 2012 Foundation Curriculum from an educational point of view, and relating this to earlier versions. Since learners must fulfil the requirements of their curriculum, the following section goes on to indicate how this can be achieved, by using principles and practice discussed throughout this book for enriching the education of the learning doctor. This enables the formal assessments to be fulfilled whilst at the same time improving them educationally, and enabling learners to accrue and place on record their own richer and more endurable evidence of their achievement.

The formal assessment 'tools' for workplace-based assessment (WPBA) in PGME

In the original 'seven pillars of MMC', assessment was set to be competency-based, and the key principles driving the 'Tools of the Trade' were that it should be: service-led; based on in-work assessment; with an open and transparent process; and be developmental and summative. Thus it was conceived as separate from teaching and learning, and was focused on competencies, with all their weaknesses. Further, the imposition of the 'Tools' was driven by the twin gods of validity and reliability, defined in highly scientific terms that were inappropriate to education, and they were also claimed to be 'research-based' whilst on inspection there was little real evidence of this and, what there was, showed the tools being used in undergraduate work and/or in other countries. They were designed to be 'feasible' which meant that they could be carried out in a few minutes, and the huge numbers of assessments to be 'collected' created a mindset that the whole process was more for the sake of collecting the badges than for any educational value.

These 'National Assessment Tools', as four assessment procedures, began development in 2003 and were finally launched for 'formal delivery nationally' in the Foundation Years, in August 2005. They have subsequently been used in, or at minimum have greatly influenced, all other medical and surgical specialties' curricula, with very little development or amendment. This is despite the fact that they were fairly simplistic and generalized even for the Foundation level, and do not really reflect much of what needs to be learnt at Core and Specialty level.

The most valuable aspect of these tools was that they established the importance of placing education (teaching, learning and assessment) in clinical practice, and replaced a haphazard approach to career advancement in which the only formal 'tests' were college written exams (which were poor indicators of sound practice), and the only other evidence for progression was the supervising consultant's opinions, often expressed informally. The idea of initiating assessments to be completed in the clinical setting, then, was good, but the processes and content of them were not universally well received and they have never quite done the job that was intended, let alone supported the educational intentions of the curriculum.

The 'tools' do not resonate well with many clinicians, while educators see them as overly narrow and behaviourist. See the front of this chapter for a 'trainee's' view in 2011, and for a consultant's version published earlier, see Talbot (2004). Both writers were speaking for many doctors. Sadly too, the very title of this collection of assessment processes as 'Tools of the Trade', implied that medicine was a trade and undermined the idea that learning doctors needed to develop their professionalism in practice. In presenting these processes as 'tools', the essentially 'technical' nature of assessment was reinforced, and this was emphasized further in the tick-list approach they adopted for reporting achievement. Their design was aimed at producing a process that could be speedily conducted in the clinical setting and by a variety of 'assessors', rather than by the clinical supervisor who knew the trainee and could chart their educational and clinical development. This was in the name of a spurious 'objectivity'. The intention was to 'prove' that the trainee had undergone the right number of processes with a mixture of examiners.

In short, these 'tools', whose very name celebrated their technical pedigree, were conceived of and driven by the narrowest of technical demands, and their only real interest was in accruing numbers of passes, irrespective of quality, and with no interest in promoting and rewarding understanding and educational development. Further, being set out separately as 'self-standing' processes that 'tested' clinical practice using a wide range of assessors, served inadvertently to undermine the supervisor/trainee relationship and the significance of education. Indeed, there is considerable evidence to show that eight years after their first appearance, they are still the only elements of the formal curriculum that many supervisors know about and that the very extensive focus on assessment has deflected the energies of teacher and learner from more educational processes.

In short the tools seem to have been far more about both teacher and learner getting through this process in the clinical setting as fast as possible (so as not to interrupt patient care), than about engaging in an educational process that generates serious evidence, on record, of the learner's achievements. Further, it is the teacher who fills in the forms and thus creates the evidence that is placed on record but does not provide details of the learner's development. This means that there is no formal opportunity for the *learner* to contribute any enduring evidence of their achievements. In principle the enhancement of such assessment, where only the teacher records evidence and that evidence is broadly numerical, is for the learner to contribute complementary evidence in words. As we shall see, this might best be done through clinical reflective writing (CRW) that illuminates the learner's thinking processes in CBD, DOPs or Mini-CEX.

Eight years later however, there has been a very little fundamental development of these processes, as the draft 2012 Foundation Curriculum reveals.

The Foundation Curriculum (2012) and how it relates to earlier versions

(Please note that this document was still in draft form as this book went to print.) In the latest version of these workplace-based assessments, the term 'tools' has finally been dropped. The new Foundation Curriculum, no doubt still leading the way for all other postgraduate medical curricula lists its modifications in Appendix D but this edition appears still redolent of earlier versions. Like them, it contains considerable over-assessment, (though there is less than before) and its narrowly technical focus still needs widening. However, it does place assessment more directly in the hands of supervisors and no longer sees it as summative.

This section, then offers a brief overview of the four formal assessment processes as proposed in the draft 2012 Foundation Curriculum.

1. Team Assessment of Behaviour (TAB) (previously called Multi-Source Feedback (MSF) and 360-degree assessment)

The newly christened TAB is the same 'multi-source feedback' process as before, which in turn was based on '360 degree assessment'. As previously, it consists of the collated views about the doctor's behaviour with or in front of colleagues. These 'raters' consist of a range of co-workers that the doctor chooses from a recommended list of appropriate post-holders (which excludes other foundation doctors). The items to be rated also map to a self-assessment tool with identical domains. This TAB normally should take place once per year, although deaneries may increase the frequency. It is suggested that it be taken in the last month of the first placement each year. This 'tool' requires the foundation doctor to nominate fifteen raters, and a minimum of ten returns is required. There is a required mix of raters which should include at least 2 of: Doctors above F2; Senior nurses above band 5; allied health professionals; other team members including ward clerks, secretaries and auxiliary staff. This is more explicit than before in specifying the role of non-medical staff. If, as before, there are concerns about any foundation doctor, the TAB can be repeated in the last four months during the year of training.

As found under earlier versions of this curriculum, this process can be a useful teaching resource where the teacher helps the 'trainee' to consider the differences (and the reasons for them) between raters and between the TAB rating and a self-rating, (though which is the more accurate may not always be clear). Although it can be repeated later in an attachment, this is usually a one-off procedure.

It should be noted however, that a number of dangers exist in using it educationally. Firstly, its focus on behaviour rather than conduct indicates that it is about only what is visible and desired by others, not what the learner understands, believes in and is committed to. Secondly, it is about how a doctor 'performs' within a team, but the assessment is not in fact focused on a particular team experience, rather on a random group who may never have worked together in a specific team to a specific end — beyond all being members of the same institution. Thirdly, it is open to a considerable range of manipulative influences because of how raters are chosen, and on what basis they engage in the process. Fourthly, it needs to be recognized in exploring the results that, ironically, good doctors commonly rate themselves below others' views of them while poorer doctors rate themselves above. Finally, being a one-off event, it has limited value in any serious educational programme, which should be about development.

2. Two assessment procedures within the supervised learning events (SLEs) in the clinical setting

The SLE is a new term. It emphasizes the importance of the assessment procedures being used in front of the supervisor. In this, it is an improvement over earlier versions which seemed to allow learners to ask for an assessment *post hoc.* There are two procedures within the SLEs that must take place in the clinical setting: the Mini-CEX, and the DOPs. There are still no changes in these processes.

The Mini-CEX is a structured assessment of an observed clinical encounter. It must not be completed after a ward round presentation or when the doctor/ patient interaction was not directly observed. Foundation doctors should complete a minimum of six Mini-CEXs in the first Foundation year (F1) and another six in the second year (F2). These should be spaced out during the year with at least two Mini-CEXs completed in each four-month period, but there is no maximum number. A different assessor should be used for each, including at least one at consultant or GP level, per four-month placement. Each Mini-CEX must represent a different clinical problem. The rater fills in a tick-list form containing also an expandable box for additional comment and advice. There is nothing fundamentally new in this process or how it is presented.

The DOPs provides 'a structured checklist for giving feedback on the foundation doctor's interaction with the patient when performing a practical procedure'. Learners may submit up to three DOPs in one year as part of the minimum requirements for evidence of observed doctor/patient encounters. Different assessors should be used for each DOPs, and each should represent a different procedure. Beyond the Foundation years, DOPs will assess procedural skills, but in these first two years only the doctor/patient interaction is focused on. There is no maximum requirement for the number of DOPs a doctor can undertake. Again, there has been no real change or development of this procedure since it was first introduced.

These two processes, that have not been conceived *educationally*, contain the following flaws:

▷ a different 'rater' is required on every occasion

▷ the areas to be rated are far too general to generate useful details of the learner's abilities and achievements

▷ the associated discussions about the assessment event are too brief to provide educationally worthwhile depth

▷ the scale on which the rater works is a skewed version of a Lickert scale (which in its purer form is used in research questionnaires)

▷ the forms privilege numbers as recorded evidence rather than words, and such numbers lose their significance over time and with multiple raters

▷ what is recorded is simplistic and without detail

▷ the main evidence used to make these decisions is what is visible

▷ the categories are only those which can be quickly captured

▷ there is no evidence from the learner on the resulting record, to balance the evidence of the forms which are both vestigial and are completed only by the teacher.

Indeed, such an approach to assessment (even where it needs to be 'work-based) would be ethically unacceptable to professional teachers, for all these reasons. Different raters (required in the spurious interests of objectivity), means no sense of continuity and no evidence of educational development. The areas to be rated are defined in no more useful terms than previously offered and use the word 'appropriate' frequently, which begs the question about how many different versions of 'appropriate' will be endemic (but untraceable) across the set of forms, in, for example, rating 'critical judgement'. Further, it seems odd to be rating the important complexities defined in this category with one rating only. In addition, the 1 to 6 scale offers too many categories. Educationally inexperienced raters will tend towards the middle range and those politically motivated to gain a generous reputation for the Trust will seek to use the top wherever possible.

On all these matters, the tick-box requirements have not changed from earlier versions of these assessment processes. There is still no chance of using the evidence from these forms to chart the continuity of the educational development of the learner (except at a very generalized level) and the judgement of each 'rater' is less than educationally reliable as they have no developmental context within which to understand the learner's achievements and progression. Indeed, these two flaws ensure that the assessment processes cannot easily provide an educational experience for the learner! Only by a department acting as a faculty and establishing a coherent and rigorous approach to reflecting on each process, could this be remedied.

3. Two assessment procedures used within the SLEs that take place remote from the patient

There are two SLEs that take place remote from the patient: the Case-based Discussion (CBD); and developing the clinical teacher.

Case based discussion is a 'structured discussion' of a clinical case that has been managed by the foundation doctor. Its 'strength' is quoted as being 'an investigation of, and feedback on, clinical reasoning' (draft Foundation Curriculum 2012: 58). This emphasis on 'clinical reasoning' is new and to be applauded, but it needs to be backed up by assessment forms that attend to such matters in more detail and by reflective processes that enable the learner to draw out the patterns and achievements of, and to offer their own personal perspectives on, their thinking.

Across the Foundation Programme, a minimum of six CBDs should be completed with at least two CBDs undertaken in any four-month period. Again, different assessors should be used for each wherever possible; assessors should have sufficient experience of the area under consideration. There is no maximum of CBDs required. The discussion involved is still expected to be brief, the learner concentrating on presenting the basic clinical details about the patient and the teacher asking further questions or giving advice.

The criticism of these processes as described earlier applies equally to the CBD as required in the curriculum.

Developing the clinical teacher is now up-fronted as the other assessment process in this kind of SLE. This involves the supervisor completing a form on the observation of a foundation doctor's presentational and teaching skills! Although not new, this seems to have been given more prominence in the way it is presented in this curriculum. I would argue strongly that such a form is an unwise part of the preparation of a doctor to be a PGME teacher. Firstly, it misleadingly brings up young doctors to see teaching only as a technical presentational process (which this book suggests is a highly impoverished view of it). Secondly, it implies that anyone can teach anyone anything, as long as they know a little more than their learners. This might be true for an experienced teacher who understands what providing an educationally worthwhile experience for the learner involves. For the inexperienced doctor, however, it seems to reinstate and give credence to the outmoded and somewhat insulting notion that all that teaching requires is to 'see one, do one and then teach one'. This whole enterprise is, arguably very dangerous, is certainly largely ineffective, and is prone to misleading the learner about the importance — for patient safety and care — of engaging in sound PGME which focuses on the educationally worthwhile, and is offered by a teacher who has gravitas and authority.

Creating and using the evidence from these assessments

The Logbook / portfolio

Electronic-portfolios (E-portfolios) are used as a means of collecting and storing the results of the assessment processes in a variety of specialties as well as in the Foundation Years. They are required for successful completion of all specialty programmes and are presented at a formal summative assessment at the end of each placement and at the end of the year. For the first Foundation Year, the GMC requires demonstration to the Foundation Lead of competence in a series of procedures, in order for a provisionally registered doctor (FI) to be eligible for full registration before entering the F2 year. Beyond the Foundation, there is an assessment panel that considers every individual portfolio and where necessary meets the candidate. Driessen (2008) and Norman (2008) debate how well such portfolios improve assessment. A critique of portfolio assessment is offered in the following section.

The reports from both the clinical and educational supervisor

Two end of placement reports are required: the clinical supervisor's and the educational supervisor's (the draft Foundation Curriculum 2012: 60). The clinical supervisor's report describes the performance of the foundation doctor in the workplace. It focuses on noteworthy aspects of the doctor's performance; any concerns about performance; details of the doctor's appropriate participation in the agreed educational process; and evidence of personal and professional development as a result of feedback and reflection. The educational supervisor's report incorporates 'the information contained in this report' and in addition includes information from the e-portfolio. The curriculum states that:

> Whilst engagement with supervised learning events (SLEs) and evidence of curriculum coverage will be taken into account, the overall judgement will include a triangulated view of the doctor's day to day work performance, which will include their participation in, and attendance at, educational activities, appraisals, the learning process and recording of this in the e-portfolio.
>
> *(Ibid: 60)*

These are important matters but it is not clear, even in the following, how they will be balanced against the evidence from the assessment procedures.

The end of year report from the educational supervisor.

Placement reports are drawn together in the educational supervisor's End of Year Report, which will form the basis of the Foundation Programme director's recommendations regarding satisfactory completion of FI and the Foundation Programme as a whole. This is an overall professional judgement of the foundation doctor. It should reflect the outcome of the final assessment discussion and should be agreed by both the foundation doctor and the educational supervisor and recorded in the doctor's e-portfolio on the "End of placement review" form.

These processes involve the educational supervisor (with the learning doctor) reviewing the evidence from colleagues, as found in the assessment forms and the portfolio. These will not provide very robust evidence as they will appear simply as ticks in boxes, whose original meaning becomes less clear once they are scrutinized somewhat later, and which only provide the crudest of patterns. This is all deeply bureaucratic and seems to require more time on form-filling and report writing than on teaching and learning! Were it more 'educationally focused', the time involved would be more worthwhile.

Given that there are clearly some educational reservations about the assessment processes as they stand at the moment, how might these be addressed?

Making these assessment processes more educational

Readers who already understand the significance of the moral mode of practice will, by now, readily perceive that the present formal assessment system for PGME is far too entrenched in the technical mode of practice alone, and will recognize the need to enrich it by using the assessment principles already explained and explored in chapters eight and eleven.

Given that we cannot change these procedures, but only add to them, clearly the principal need here is to balance the current generalized, numerical, and technical focus, which is interested in learners' skills and knowledge, by something that attends to their education in respect of their conduct, character and understanding, as found in their being, knowing, doing, thinking and becoming.

The current assessment processes that offer the best potential for this are the Mini-CEX, the DOPs and the CBD. For ways of seating the teaching of a procedure in the moral rather than the technical mode of practice and the resulting change in the nature of the assessment, see above, pp. 151-53. For ways of enriching the CBD see the Case-based Discussion Plus process (CbD Plus ©) button on www. ED4MEDPRAC.co.uk, and the Clinical Reflective Writing (CRW) button.

For these separated assessment encounters to become a fully integrated part of the education of junior doctors, the portfolio structure and content need to be further developed (see the final section of this chapter).

The following principles and practice would build *quality* into the PGME formal assessment processes by making them more educational.

▷ Assessment should be embedded within the teaching and learning process, not appear to run alongside it. Thus the clinical supervisor should be more fully a part of the assessment process.

▷ Assessment should be carried out by those who know about and understand the learner's progress and development (those who teach them), and not by a series of one-off encounters with those outside the educational process.

▷ In the clinical setting, any summative assessment should use multiple perspectives to understand practice from as many points of view as possible. Such multiple perspectives should take account of:

- the visible performance of the learner
- the learner's ability to articulate the driving forces underpinning their clinical performance
- how the learner's ideas, beliefs, values and assumptions have influenced their performance
- the impact of the learner's performance on all others involved
- how the learner has used the learning opportunities provided

- the quality of their self-knowledge
- how the learner has related theory and practice
- how much input there has been from their supervisor
- how the resulting judgements compare with those made of the learner by others who teach them.

▷ In the clinical setting, assessment needs to respect the holistic nature of professional practice and not atomise it into skills alone, which though necessary are not sufficient.

▷ This requires the recognition that there is far more to clinical practice than what is visible.

▷ The record should incorporate evidence from learners' writing of their achievements, progress and ability at self-assessment, alongside their supervisor's evidence. This can be achieved by both teacher and learner engaging orally and then in writing with the reflective processes that have been designed especially for doctors looking at clinical events by using The Invisibles (see Fish and de Cossart 2007) and CRW (see website).

By this means, and particularly by the use of reflective writing, such assessment shows the quality of the learner's thinking and clinical expertise. Such reflection:

▷ should strive to honour the real complexity of clinical settings and the richness of detail which affect intelligent practice within them

▷ should consider how the learner has used the opportunities available for learning. The scope of the opportunities available should be considered during assessment, in order to be fair about what can be expected from the learner, given the nature of the practice context

▷ must be valid and reliable, *in educational terms,* since assessment is a form of educational inquiry. This uses qualitative research procedures to investigate the complexity of lived experience. A more educational view of validity and reliability is as follows.

Validity of assessment procedures in an educational context means checking that a variety of assessment processes are used both within the assessment of a practical process and across the practice as a whole and that these do justice to its complexity and are represented in the final assessment. This involves the use of multiple perspectives (sometimes also called 'triangulation'). *Consequential validity* asks whether worthwhile and effective learning has taken place as a result of the assessment.

Reliability in an educational context means the assessment will assess that which it sets out to do, and not, (by accident) some other element. This involves teacher and learner in being clear about, and agreeing to, what is being assessed and how, and that these are appropriate to the context chosen for the assessment.

The importance of reflection

In all there are 15 references to reflection in the draft 2012 Foundation Curriculum, but nowhere is there any help with how to reflect. A typical example is:

> Foundation doctors should reflect on and learn from their positive and negative experiences in order to demonstrate clinical development.
>
> *Foundation Curriculum 2012, pp. 11*

Good clinical reflection for doctors is at last beginning to be recognized as the essential core of worthwhile PGME, but it requires careful nurturing and thorough understanding. Further, the reflective practice approach used by non-medical healthcare practitioners is not suitable for doctors seeking to learn from their clinical events and encounters. In short, reflection for doctors is not the simple activity it has been taken for (and if mistreated as such will not yield the important educational enlightenment that it should bring). It is highly important both for doctors who are developing well (in order to explore and record their growing expertise) and for learners in difficulty (in order to pinpoint, diagnose and attend to their clinical shortfall).

For help with this from a well-researched and experienced source, readers should seek out the current and shortly to be published work of Fish and de Cossart, and examples of CRW as offered on their website.

The significance of portfolios: some ideas for the future

In any more 'root and branch' attempt to improve the current assessment procedures, the portfolio will be an important component, and so this final section explores its possibilities. Teachers and learners in PGME thus need to think about how else they could use the portfolio, beyond the currently given, and rather narrowly conceived, purposes and sections.

Portfolios can fulfil a range of different intentions within a general broad aim to provide readers (assessors and others) with evidence of the development of a learner's understanding and achievements. One approach might be developed by learner and teacher *together* selecting samples of best work which has already been responded to by the supervisor and which has been divided into mandated or chosen sections, in order to demonstrate evidence of (final) achievement. A second approach might be for the learner to present samples of unmarked work that the learner believes show their progression throughout a course or attachment, which shows growth of various kinds. Its intention would be to provide teachers, learners and others with reason to be interested, with evidence of progression, and to submit this evidence to the teacher for their final judgement. Each section would need to be brought together with some kind of summary overview to enable a final judgement to be made about the quality of the learning (and perhaps about the learner's readiness to progress to another level). In some courses, a portfolio of coursework becomes an appendix as evidence to be drawn upon in a written assignment, which forms the main part of the assessed work.

Clearly, the focus of the different sections is significant, as is how these are brought together by the learner to offer a cohesive presentation. Used well the portfolio can contain a wide variety of different kinds of assessment that assess different perspectives (and it is this variety that needs to be enriched in PGME). Also the strategies used to help the learner compile *and own* the evidence are interesting. At a technical level, this includes keeping abreast of the progress over time and not assuming it can all be left until the end. At an educational level, it is about helping learners to focus on how the assessment has *promoted* learning as well as checked up on it.

There are some interesting issues that are worth discussing with learners as they collect evidence and use the portfolio educationally. These include the following questions.

▷ To what extent is a portfolio actually 'a performance'?

▷ How far does (or should) it reflect the efforts of the teacher as well as the learner?

▷ Should portfolios represent a *coached* performance?

▷ Should they be shared more between peers, and if so, what would be the educational benefits and the disadvantages ?

▷ Should we, then, in the portfolio, expect to recognize and acknowledge the profit we have had from the assistance of others?

▷ Should we expect other learners to review, help, critique our portfolios?

▷ Should there be a viva for the portfolio? Indeed, who should review and assess the portfolio, and should the learner be present during this?

But the biggest question for PGME is: how can we make the portfolios required in medicine *more alive* and more about real evidence of learning in practice?

As this chapter has shown, then, if treated educationally, the assessment processes discussed could be the basis of the sound development of (and the generation of robust evidence of) the learning doctor's educational achievements.

Last words

This book has presented an in-depth illustration of what can be achieved within PGME when it is focused on the moral mode of practice and engaged in by teachers who understand what is involved in worthwhile education. It provides this material as a contribution to serious national debate about the future aims, aspirations and quality of PGME, and as evidence of what can be achieved in terms of the enhancement of the teaching, learning and assessment that doctors both need and deserve at the local level.

The final words, however, belong to the cohort of the Chester University PG Cert with whom this book began. The quality of their educational thinking and understanding resulting from the course has been captured by a short quotation from their work at Diploma level as recorded in *Frame 12.1 Educational* praxis *in action*, as follows. It will be noted that these extracts show the writers' awareness of the complexities and challenges of educational practice and their recognition that any response to these are context specific. All members of this cohort are employees of The Countess of Chester NHS Foundation Trust, Chester, UK. Some (as indicated additionally) also work in other Merseyside hospitals. The frame concludes with the words of a learner, which typify the kinds of response regularly received by these teachers.

Frame 12.1 Educational *praxis* in action

Allowing the learner freedom during the session meant that we deviated from the proposed plan. He started talking about the consent process with children and it became clear that he has some mis-perceptions about the regulations surrounding this. Again, this was something that was essential to correct immediately. It meant that I didn't complete all my agenda item; I made an educational judgement that this was appropriate in this case.

> Miss Katharine Fleming, Consultant in Oral and
> Maxillofacial surgery at Aintree Hospital
> and the Countess of Chester Hospital

On this occasion [as the teacher] I was going to have to juggle a number of conflicting aspects ... how would I allow for true thinking without "socking it to him"? How would I be able to teach in the moral mode of practice ... for the sake of the longer-term goal?

> Dr Natalie Meara, Consultant Histopathologist

I should not be surprised, but I did not realize how much my initial plan [for a teaching session] would change as I learnt more about myself and my learner... the old me would have been fairly flexible, but I don't think I would have had the knowledge and confidence to make some of the changes I did.... The old Latin saying: '*Qui docet dixit*' (he who teaches learns) is me!

> Ann Baker, Clinical Education Manager

Previously I would have seen: 'What did I teach him?' and 'What did he learn?' as essentially interchangeable.... My educational philosophy has now shifted to one centred around the learner — how can I help them think, how can I help them to explore new areas for themselves, how can I awaken the "learner within"?

> Dr Nick Laundy, Consultant in Emergency Medicine
> and Foundation Training Programme Director

By their very nature, however, training courses [like those on 'Breaking Bad News'] which inculcate set behaviours [sic] cannot truly prepare doctors to sensitively deal with such unique, important and challenging patient interactions. Therefore not only for reasons of safe patient care, but also for increased patient satisfaction, it is imperative that we, as doctors, undergo self-exploration of our practice, and through considered reflection draw upon our findings to enhance our future practice [educational and clinical].

Dr Jamie Fanning, Specialty Doctor in Anaesthesia
And Critical Care Medicine

Current Medical Education includes significant emphasis on the virtues of evidence. In contrast there is little if any time devoted to the evidence of virtue. At times a moral practitioner must *dare* to be wise. Wisdom is seen as a virtue that requires daring. Kant showed that wisdom was a determined independence to be morally good. We need to bring our educational practice closer to this.

Dr Eileen Fantom, Associate Specialist in Emergency Medicine

The powerful impression people have in influencing my character, in re-configuring me as a person and me as a doctor has allowed me to see, deliberately form and refine what works for me. It provides me comfort when I struggle to be the person that I am. He [The learner] has matured.... He feels his character has developed considerably more now that he is comfortable with his own medical knowledge, but it is the identifying and recognizing the importance of his character that has given him a focus that is not purely based on medicine.

Dr Ian Benton, Consultant Respiratory Physician

I struggled with thinking of strategies for how to stimulate him [the learner] to break out of his cycle .... In fact, it was only when writing myself that the idea came to me for putting the learner in the position of a senior doctor .... Clearly the discovery of a blind-spot in the learner's knowledge or thinking needs to be addressed sensitively .... As a teacher I realize that it is important to consider how to respond when his [the learner's response] isn't what you had entirely hoped for.

Mr David Monk, Consultant General and Upper
Gastrointestinal Surgeon

The session was more of an equal professional conversation, a joint enquiry via exploratory talk, to promote collective thinking, develop reasoning and understanding, with both parties listening, responding and ... building onto each other's contributions.

Dr Lyndsay Cheater: Consultant in Anaesthethesia
And Critical Care Medicine

The following verbatim oral comment from a learner sums up many of the comments learners have made:

"These sessions were completely different. We had to do something. In other sessions they just teach and we just learn half the time and half the time we are sleeping. I have never been to anything like these sessions before. We looked at ourselves and [at] how to improve you as a person ... not just [at] theory. We could discuss things — it was not just 'this is right or that is wrong', it was more of a discussion and finding different solutions, which is a good thing."

Provided by Renate Thomé, Clinical Education
Consultant and Evaluator

The Appendix

Appendix: the classical and Tomist virtues

How can we develop a virtues-based rather than a competencies-based curriculum for doctors?

(NOTE: the current four virtues listed by the GMC are: justice; autonomy; beneficence and non-maleficence)

Aristotle's virtues (The natural moral virtues ascertainable by reason and improved by practice)	Aquinas's virtues (supernatural moral virtues, infused in us by God, possessed through grace)	New Testament Matthew 22: 36 - 39
Courage	Courage	When asked: Master which is the great commendment in the law?,
Generosity	Generosity of spirit	
Fidelity to trust	Faith	
Compassion	Charity in action, *Agapé*	Jesus said unto him: 'Thou shalt love the Lord
Prudential judgement (*Phronesis*)	Prudence	with all thy heart and with all thy soul and with all thy mind.
Temperance	Temperance	This is the first and great commandment.
Justice	Charitable Justice	And second is like unto it: Thou shalt love thy neighbour as thyself.
Fortitude	Hope	On these two
Integrity	United by religious commitment?	commandments hang all
Self effacement	Humility	the law and the prophets

See also: Pellegrino and Thomasma (1993) and (1996).

References

Alexander, R. (2004) *Towards Dialogic Teaching*. Cambridge: Dialogos.

Aristotle (1925) *The Nicomachean Ethics*. Oxford: Oxford University Press.

Armstrong, J. (1996) *Looking at Pictures: An introduction to the Appreciation of Art*. London: Duckworth Press.

Barnes, D. (1995) The Role of Talk in Learning, in K. Norman (ed) *Thinking Voices: The work of the National Oracy Project*. London: Hodder & Stoughton.

Barrow, R. (2002) Or What's a heaven for? In R. Marples (ed) *The Aims of Education*. London: Routledge.

Benjamin, H. (1939) The sabre-tooth Curriculum, in M. Golby, J. Greenwald, and R. West, (eds) (1975) *Curriculum Design*. London: Croom Helm in Association with Open University press.

Bolton, G. (2010) *Reflective Practice: Writing and Professional Development*. London: Sage Publications (Third Edition).

Boud, D., Keogh, R. and Walker, D. (1985) *Reflection: Turning Experience into Learning*. London: Sage Publications.

Bondi, E., Carr, D., Clark, C. and Clegg, C. (eds) (2010) *Towards Professional Wisdom: Practical Deliberation in the People Professions*. Farnham, Surrey: Ashgate.

Broadfoot, P. (1996) Educational Assessment: The myth of measurement, in P. Woods (ed) *Contemporary Issues in teaching and learning*. London: RoutledgeFalmer.

Brown, L.M. (1970) *Aims of Education*. New York: Teachers College Press.

Bullock, A., Hardyman, J. and Phillips, S. (2012) *Quality Teaching and Learning in clinical practice for F2 Teachers and Learners:* Cardiff: Cardiff University.

Cameron, D. (2001) *Working With Spoken Discourse*. London: Sage Publications.

Carr, D. (1993) Questions of Competence, *British Journal of Educational Studies*, **41**: 253-271.

Carr, D. (2000) *Professionalism and Ethics in Teaching*. London: Routledge.

Carr, D. (2003) *Making Sense of Education: An introduction to the philosophy and theory of education and teaching*. London: RoutledgeFalmer.

Carr, D. (2004) Rival Conceptions of Practice in Education and Teaching, in J. Dunne and P. Hogan (eds) *Education and Practice: Upholding the Integrity of Teaching and Learning*. Oxford: Blackwell Publishing.

Carr, D. (2005a) Personal and interpersonal relationships in education and teaching: a virtue ethical perspective, *British Journal of Educational Studies*, **53** (3): 255-271.

Carr, D. (2005b) On the contribution of literature and the arts to the educational cultivation of moral virtue, feeling and emotion, *Journal of Moral Education*, **34** (2): 137-151.

Carr, D. (2006) Professional and personal values and virtues in education and teaching, *Oxford Review of Education*, **32** (2): 171-183.

Carr, D. (2007) Character in Teaching, *British Journal of Educational Studies*, **55** (4): 369-389.

Carr, W. (1995) What is an Educational Practice? *For Education: Towards Critical Educational Enquiry*. Buckingham: Open University Press.

Carr, W. (2009) A Postmodern Perspective on Professional Practice, in B. Green (ed) *Understanding and Researching Professional Practice*. Rotterdam: Sense Publications.

Cruess, R.L., Cruess, S.R., and Steinert, Y. (2008) *Medical Professionalism*. Cambridge: Cambridge University Press.

de Cossart, L. and Fish, D. (2005) *Cultivating a Thinking Surgeon: new perspectives on clinical teaching, learning and assessment*. Shrewsbury: TfN Publications.

de Cossart, L. and Fish, D. (2012) Clinical Reflection: The Heart of Continuing Professional Development for Doctors, *Medical Women, 31* (1): 10-11

Dent, J.A., and Harden, R.M. (eds) (2009) *A Practical Guide for Medical Educators*. Edinburgh: Elsevier.

Dijkstra, J., Van der Vleuten, C.P., and Schuwirth, L.W. (2009). A new framework for designing programmes of assessment, *Advanced Health Science Education: Theory and Practice*.

Dobson, S., Dobson, M. and Bromley, L. (2011) *How to teach: A Handbook for Clinicians*. Oxford: Oxford University Press.

Dornan, T., Mann, K., Scherpbier, A. and Spencer, J. (2011) *Medical Education: Theory and Practice*. London: Churchill Livingstone / Elsevier.

Downey, R. (1999) The role of Literature in Medical Education: A commentary on the poem: Roswell, Hanger 84, *Journal of Medical Ethics* **25**: 529 – 31.

Driessen, E. (2008) Are Learning portfolios worth the effort? Yes, *British Medical Journal, **337***: 320

Dunne, J. (1995) *Back to the Rough Ground*. Paris: Notre Dame Press.

Dunne, J. (2005) An Intricate Fabric: understanding the rationality of practice, *Pedagogy, Culture and Society, **13*** (3): 367-89

Dunne, J. and Hogan P. (2004) Introduction, in J. Dunne and P. Hogan (eds) *Education and Practice: Upholding the Integrity of Teaching and Learning*. Oxford: Blackwell Publishers.

Eliot. T.S. Burnt Norton, *Collected poems* 1909-35. London: Faber and Faber.

Evans, D. (2001) Imagination and Medical Education, *Journal of Medical Ethics*, **27**: 30-34.

Fish, D. (1998) *Appreciating Practice in the Caring Professions*. Oxford: Heinemann.

Fish, D. (2010) Learning to practise Interpretively: exploring and developing practical rationality, in J. Higgs, D. Fish, I. Goulter, S. Loftus, J-A. Reid and F. Trede (eds) *Education for Future Practice*. Rotterdam: Sense Publications: 191-202.

Fish, D. and Brigley, S. (2010) 'Exploring the Practice of Education' in J. Higgs, D. Fish, I. Goulter, S. Loftus, J-A. Reid and F. Trede (eds), *Education for Future Practice*. Rotterdam: Sense Publications, 113-122.

Fish, D. and Coles, C. (2005) *Medical Education: Developing a Curriculum for Practice*. Maidenhead:

Open University Press.

Fish, D. and de Cossart, L. (2007), *Developing the Wise Doctor*. London: Royal Society of Medicine Press.

Freire, P. (1970) *Pedagogy of the Oppressed*. London: Penguin Books.

Freire, P. (1998/2001) *Pedagogy of Freedom: Ethics, Democracy, and Civic Courage*. Oxford: Rowman and Littlefield Publishers Inc.

General Medical Council (2006) *Good Medical Practice*. London: GMC.

Golby, M. (1993) Educational Research: Trick or Treat? *Exeter Society for Curriculum Studies*, **15**: (3): 5-8.

Golby, J. and Parrott, A. (2002) *Educational Practice and Educational Research*. Tiverton: Fair Way Press.

Grundy, S. (1987) *Curriculum: Product or Praxis*. London: The Falmer Press.

Gunderman, R.B. (2006) *Achieving Excellence in Medical Education*. New York: Springer.

Habermas, J. (1974) *Theory and Practice*. London: Heinemann.

Hansen, D. (2001) *Exploring the Moral Heart of Teaching: Towards a Teacher's Creed*. New York: Teachers College Press.

Hirst, P. and Peters, R. S. (1970) *The Logic of Education*. London: Routledge.

Hunter, K. M. (1991) *Doctors' Stories: The Narrative Structure of Medical Knowledge*. Princeton, NJ: Princeton University Press.

Iliffe, S. (2008) *From General Practice to Primary Care: The Industrialization of Family Medicine*. Oxford: Oxford University Press.

Jacklin, R., Sevdalis, N., Harries, C., Darzi, A., Vincent, C. (2008). Judgment analysis: a method for quantitative evaluation of trainee surgeons' judgments of surgical risk. *American Journal of Surgery*, **195**: 183-188.

Jackson, N., Jamieson, A. and Khan, A. (eds) (2007) *Assessment in Medical Education and Training: a practical guide*. Oxford: Radcliffe Publishing.

Jessup, G. (1991) *Outcomes: Nvqs And The Emerging Model of Education and Training*. London: Falmer Press.

Kee, F., McDonald, P., Kirwan, J. R., Patterson, C.C., Love, A.H.G. (1998) Urgency and priority for cardiac surgery: a clinical judgment analysis., *British Medical Journal*, **316**: 925-929.

Kemmis, S. and Smith T.J. (eds) (2008) *Enabling Praxis: Challenges for Education*. Rotterdam: Sense Publishers.

Kemmis, S. and Smith, T.J. (2008) Chapter One: Personal Praxis, S. Kemmis and T.J. Smith (eds) *Enabling Praxis: Challenges for Education*. Rotterdam: Sense Publishers.

Kenny, N. and Shelton, W. (eds) (2006) *Lost Virtue: Professional Character Development in Medical Education* (Advances in Bioethics Volume 10). Amsterdam: Elsevier JAI.

Longley, C. (2010) Thought for the Day: 8th February 2010: BBC.

Lieberman A. and Miller L. (eds) (2008) *Teachers in professional communities: Improving teaching and learning.* New York: Teachers College Press.

Macklin, R. (2009) Moral Judgement and Practical Reasoning in professional practice, in B. Green (ed) *Understanding and Researching Professional Practice.* Rotterdam: Sense Publications.

MacCormack, A.D. and Parry, B.R. (2006) Judgment analysis of surgeons' prioritisation of patients for elective general surgery, *Medical Decision Making,* **26**: 255.

MacLure, M. (2003) *Discourse in Educational and Social Research.* Buckingham: Open University Press.

Mann, K. (2006) Learning and Teaching in Professional Character Development, in N. Kenny and W. Shelton eds) *Lost Virtue: Professional Character Development in Medical Education* (Advances in Bioethics Volume 10). Amsterdam: Elsevier JAI.

Marples, R. (ed) (1999) *The Aims of Education* (Routledge International Studies in Philosophy). London: Routledge.

Meara, N. and Guiliani, K. (2011) How do we measure Learning? *The Bulletin of The Royal College of Pathologists,* **156**: 255-58.

Mercer, N. (1995/ 2008) *The Guided Construction of Knowledge: talk amongst teachers and learners.* Bristol: Multilingual Matters Ltd.

Mercer, N. (2000) *Words and Minds: How we use language to think together.* London: Routledge.

Montgomery, K. (2006) *How Doctors Think: clinical judgement and the practice of medicine.* Oxford: Oxford University Press.

Moon, J. (1999) *Reflection in Learning and Personal development: Theory and Practice.* London: RoutledgeFalmer.

Neuberger, J. (2006) *The Moral State We're In: A manifesto for the 21st Century.* London: HarperCollinsPublishers.

Norman, G. (2008) Are Learning Portfolios worth the effort? No. *British Medical Journal,* **337**: 321.

Norman, K. (ed) (1995) *Thinking Voices: The work of the National Oracy Project.* London: Hodder & Stoughton.

Oakeshott, M. (1967) Learning and Teaching, in R.S. Peters (ed), *The Concept of Education.* London: Routledge and Kegan Paul.

O' Neill, O. (2002) *A Question of Trust: The BBC Reith Lectures.* Cambridge: Cambridge University Press.

Palmer, Parker, J. (1998) *The Courage to Teach.* San Francisco: Jossey Bass.

Passmore, J. (1981) *The Philosophy of Teaching.* London: Duckworth Press.

Pellegrino, E.D. (2006) Character Formation and the making of good physicians, in N. Kenny and W. Shelton (eds) *Lost Virtue: Professional Character Development in Medical Education* (Advances in Bioethics Volume 10). Amsterdam: Elsevier JAI.

Pellegrino, E.D. and Thomasma, D.C. (1993) *The Virtues in Medical Practice.* Oxford: Oxford University Press.

Pellegrino, E.D. and Thomasma, D.C. (1996) *The Christian Virtues in Medical Practice.* Washington DC: Georgetown University Press.

Peters, R.S. (1966) *Ethics and Education.* London: Unwin University Books.

Phenix, P. (1964) *Realms of Meaning.* New York: McGraw-Hill.

Pollock, A.M. (2004) *NHS plc: the Privatisation of our Health Care.* London: Verso.

Popper, K. R. (2002) *Conjectures and Refutations.* London: Routledge.

Quirk, M. (2006) *Intuition and Metacognition in Medical Education: Keys to developing expertise.* New York: Springer Publishing Company

Schama, S. (1996), The Flaubert of the Trenches. *New Yorker,* April 1st pp. 97-8.

Schön, D. (1987) *Educating the Reflective Practitioner.* New York: Jossey Bass.

Seddon, J. (2008) *Systems Thinking in the Public Sector.* London: Triarchy Press.

Seldon, A. (2009) *Trust: How We Lost It And How To Get It Back.* London: Backbite Publishing.

Sevdalis, N. and Jacklin, R. (2008) Opening the "Black box" of surgeons' risk estimation: From intuition to quantitative modeling. *World Journal of Surgery,* **32**: (1): 324-325.

Smith, R. (1992) Theory: an entitlement to understanding, *Cambridge Journal of Education,* **22**: (3): 386-398.

Standish, P. (1999) Education without Aims? In Marples, R. (ed) *The Aims of Education* (Routledge International Studies in Philosophy). London: Routedge: 35-50.

Stenhouse, L. (1975) *An Introduction to Curriculum Research and Development.* London: Heinemann.

Talbot, M. (2004) 'Monkey see, monkey do: a critique of the competency model in graduate medical education. *Medical Education,* **38** (6): 587-92. http://www.ncbi.nlm.nih.gov/pubmed/15189254.

Thomé, R. (2012) *Educational Practice Development: An evaluation (An exploration of the impact on participants and their shared organistion of a Postgraduate Certificate in Education for Postgraduate Medical Practice 2010-2011).* Chester: Countess of Chester Hospital.

Trilling, L. (1950) Manners, morals and the novel, in *The Liberal Imagination,* New York: New York Review of Books.

Tripp, D. (1993) *Critical Incidents in Teaching: Developing Professional Judgement.* London: Routledge.

Veatch, R.M. (2006) Character Formation in Professional Education: a word of caution, in N. Kenny and W.Shelton (eds) *Lost Virtue: Professional Character Development in Medical Education* (Advances in Bioethics Volume 10). Amsterdam: Elsevier JAI.

Wells, G. (1992) The Centrality of talk in Education, in K. Norman (ed) *Thinking Voices: The work of the National Oracy Project.* London: Hodder & Stoughton.

Wells, G. (1999) *Dialogic Enquiry: Towards the Sociocultural Practice and Theory of Education.* Cambridge: Cambridge University Press.

Wells, G. (2009), *The Meaning Makers: Learning to Talk and Talking to Learn*. Bristol: Multilingual Matters, 2nd Edition.

Wenger, E. (1998) *Communities of Practice: Learning, meaning and identity*. Cambridge: Cambridge University Press.

White, J. (1982) *The Aims of Education Restated*. London: Routledge and Kegan Paul.

Whitehead, A.N. (1932) *The Aims of Education and other Essays*. London: Benn.

Wilson, P.S. (1971) *Interest and Discipline in Education*. London: Routledge and Kegan Paul.

Index

absent themes (13, 18)
Academy of Medical Educators (8)
Acquinas, Thomas (72, 205)
affective factors (187)
agent
    educational (35, 39, 67)
    someone else's (32, 39)
aims
    aims, goals and ends (81)
    clarity about, and their rationale (139)
    do we need them? (83)
    educational (see educational aims)
    ends or goals (59, 80)
    of this book (7)
    of various authors (78)
    sound educational aims (85, 155)
ambulatory settings (162)
appraisal, definition (75, 121)
appropriation (113, 170)
Aristotle (35, 40, 53, 67, 99-101, 108, 110, 111, 142)
Aristotle's virtues (98, 205)
Arts, the (37, 101, 102, 105, 108, 173)
assessment
    a coherent system of (125)
    as central to teaching and learning (176)
    as a means of promoting learning (120, 124)
    choices available (182)
    definition/s of (74, 119, 121)
    educational role of (119, 123, 189)
    enriched informal (175)
    final (119, 125, 180, 196, 198)
    formal assessment (see a also Tools of the Trade)
    formal tests (college exams) (190)
    formal assessment enriched (189)
    formal formative (180, 183, 186-8)
    formal summative (119, 187, 195)
    formative (131, 183, 186-8)
    formative, definition of (176)
    informal and formal (8, 138, 175, 177)
    informal, created by the teacher (177)
    informal: educational purposes of (162, 181-3)
    informal: examples of the design of (175, 184)
    judgement in (15, 180)
    making assessment more educational (197)
    motivating (176)
    one-off assessment (125)
    principles of assessment (176, 181)
    principles that build quality into assessment (197)
    patterns of learner's achievements (125)
    portfolios (see portfolios)
    professional judgement and (122, 180)
    role of (8, 120, 131, 132, 181)
    stark warning about (177)
    summative (119, 131, 149, 153, 175-7, 180, 186, 187, 195, 197)
    summative, a definition of (176)
    tyranny of (123, 183)
    validity and reliability of (198)
authority, teacher's (73, 154)

behaviour (30, 32, 46, 49, 52, 53, 59, 60, 63, 66, 67, 74, 92, 110, 115, 121, 123, 127-9, 132, 143, 153, 163, 192)
biological model of education (85, 145)

capacity /ies (9, 23, 25, 28, 36, 51, 54, 56, 60, 80, 89, 101, 107, 111, 123, 126-28, 130, 132)

Case Based Discussion (101, 195)
CBD (189, 191, 194, 195, 197)
Case-based Discussion Plus © (197)
character (7)
    cultivation of (36, 100)
    morally good (99)
    of personality (99)
    qualities of (73, 86, 99, 100, 110)
characteristics of a good teacher / doctor (18, 20, 36, 50, 63, 64, 68, 71-4, 98, 142, 153)
category mistake (75, 122, 130)
Chester University (14, 201)
clinical reflective writing (117, 173, 191, 197)
create/ creative / creativity (5, 6, 18, 21, 22, 24, 36, 48, 54, 55, 59, 78, 81, 84, 87, 88, 95, 101, 107, 109, 112, 113, 119, 120, 129, 133, 143, 144-46, 151, 170, 175, 180-4, 186-8, 191)
creatively (18, 36, 59, 143, 186)
codified rules (89)
coming to know oneself (97)
common sense (18, 32, 49)
community of practice (25, 45, 48, 49)
compassionate intelligence (160)
competence,
    approach (130)
    definition (126)
    a holistic notion (128)
competencies (4, 46, 50, 51, 53, 72, 79, 86, 89, 126-8, 139, 142, 190),
    definition of (126)
    a number of skills (128)
competencies and capacities (89)
competency, definition (106)
competence-based approach (129)
competency-based teaching (72)
common heritage (82)
conduct (7, 35, 45, 52-4, 57, 58-60, 66-71, 81, 86, 93, 94, 99, 110, 111, 115, 127, 128, 129, 132, 139, 143, 144, 153, 157, 160, 163, 192, 197)
Confusius (70)
conversation (15, 16, 54, 68, 93, 94, 96, 110, 114, 115, 143, 152, 159, 162-5, 167, 169, 185, 187, 202)
    a key vehicle for education (143, 164)
    (see also Language)
conversational interaction, rich (162)

Countess of Chester NHS Foundation Trust (201)
credo (144) (see also personal philosophy)
critical appreciation (94, 105)
curriculum
     process model (109, 112, 150)
     product model (108, 109, 150)
     research model (109, 112, 148, 150)
     studies (108)

debate
     about quality in PGME (7)
     the aims of PGME (80)
     nature/nurture (see nature)
Deaneries (3, 16, 192)
Deliberation, effective professional (100)
deontology (66)
differentiation, importance of (147, 150)
distance, respectful (160)
Direct Observation of Procedures (101)
DOPs (101, 131, 191, 193)

Edu-action (28, 29, 31, 32, 38, 39, 156)
Educational
     aims (8, 16, 47, 70, 71, 75, 77-87, 123, 141, 143, 144, 155, 166)
     aims and intentions or objectives (75)
     aims, logic of (77, 79)
     ends (66, 83, 84, 88, 92, 147, 162)
     evaluation. definition of (74, 75)
     intentions (36, 68, 80, 82, 84, 86, 144-6, 191)
     interactions (140, 169, 177, 181)
     judgement (20, 84, 137, 146, 150, 153, 154, 180, 201)
     managerial overview (140)
     programme (123, 127, 140, 179, 180, 182, 193)
     philosophy, own (79, 137, 138, 157)
     practice, development of (156)
     principles (5, 9, 14, 89, 137, 141)
     relationships (143, 159, 160)
     theory, nature of (103-6)
     supervisor (see supervisor)
     understanding (6, 7, 9, 13, 14, 16, 22, 25, 28, 35, 39, 95, 124, 155, 176)
     values, see values
     vision, see vision
educationally worthwhile (6, 8, 31, 36, 37, 39, 58, 68, 69, 78, 82, 84, 87, 88, 93, 96, 103, 115, 123, 124, 132, 137, 138, 140-3, 151, 154, 155, 159, 164, 176, 187, 190, 194, 195)
     ends (58, 60, 68, 84, 87, 132)
     four main principles (159)
emancipation (53)
empirical disciplines (108)
ends, aims or goals (59) (also see virtuous)
epistemology / epistemological / epistemologically (51, 139, 155)
ethical
     and moral, definition of (65)
     principles (142, 160)
     rules (86)
evaluating teaching (74, 155)

evidence-based medicine (55)

firms (3, 6, 7, 95)
flourishing,
     human (28, 98, 106, 160)
     life (33, 99)
focused reflection (97)
Foundation Curriculum (101, 189-192, 195, 196, 199)
     End of placement and end of year reports (196)
     Logbook and portfolio (195)
     References to reflection (199)
     Supervised learning events (SLEs) (193)
     remote from the patient (194)
     Team assessment of behaviour (TAB) (192)
     Workplace-based assessment (189, 190, 192)

General Medical Council (8, 89)
Good Medical Practice
good practice (46, 50, 51, 87, 97)
good teacher, inner character of (73)
good teaching (7, 19, 60, 71-3, 142, 157)
     enduring traditions of (71)
Grand Theory of education (104)
growth metaphor (88)

heart and soul, personal transformation of (74, 142)
holy ground (160)

Iceberg of professional practice (101)
identity (73)
imagination, exercising of (101)
integrity (8, 69, 73, 139, 205)
Intersubjective understanding (113, 170)
instrumentalist view (20)
Instrumentalised (30)
intuition (20, 54, 80, 109, 177)
Intelligent Kindness (4, 142, 160)

Know: coming to know (misapprehensions) (97, 178)
knowledge
     co-construction of (113, 114)
Language (see also talk)
     Asking authentic questions (167)
     dialogue (70, 152, 154, 159, 162, 165, 167)
     discourse in the clinical setting (102)
     discussion (7, 13, 15-18, 23, 24, 37, 47, 49, 58, 65, 66, 86, 93, 101, 113, 115, 139, 140, 150, 160, 163-8, 173, 181, 194-6, 202)
     dialogic teaching (165, 166)
     education is mediated through (170)
     Importance of as the vehicle for (159)

Interactive pace and cognitive pace (167)
Interaction with learner/s (73, 78, 91, 112, 113, 139, 143, 146, 150, 163-7, 169-71, 181-2, 187)
Listening skills (167)
Language in Education approach (102, 112, 162)
presentational monologue (162)
role of in learning (158, 159, 162)
tone of voice and register (167)
wait time and engaging with the answer (167)
learnt helplessness (5)
Learner,
centred (161)
challenge the (176, 183)
diagnosing ... the learner (161, 175, 178-9)
extend learning (176, 181, 183)
studying the (82, 91, 159)
key agent in the learning process (131)
learner's
needs and interests (see needs)
oral engagement (155)
reflection on themselves as doctors (159)
learner/s
as a whole person (91, 92, 94, 95, 97, 98, 141)
bored (21)
commitment to (142, 160)
serving the learner (142, 160)
unfolding from within (82)
learning
agreement (81, 97, 98, 182, 185)
an impoverished and outmoded view of (44)
behaviourist view of (112)
constructivist view of (112)
continuity of (156)
definitions of (110)
enriched (159)
methods for enhancing (156)
outcomes (78, 88, 125, 145, 151)
portfolio (see portfolio)
principles for improving (169)
process (84, 109, 120, 131, 147, 150, 155, 156, 169, 179, 183, 196, 197)
socio-cultural view of (112)
theories (92)
lingua franca of the professional teacher (162)
literature and art/The Arts (36, 108, 201, 202)
managers (101)
mindful alertness (161)
mindset in the medical world (116)
Mini-Clinical Examination (131)
Mini-CEX (131, 191, 193, 197)
Modernising Medical Careers (1, 3)
Seven pillars of (190)
Modes of practice (44, 59, 60, 78, 131, 132, 153)
Models of teaching

Product model (150)
Process Model (150)
Research Model (109, 150)
moral
agent (7)
awareness (7, 51, 73, 87, 89, 110, 142)
compass (51, 98)
dimensions (54, 155)
imperatives (5)
sensibility (27, 71, 101, 160)
sensibility and authority (71)
tradition (70)
morally
sound teachers (71)
good character (99)
Morbidity and Mortality meeting (168)
motivation of teachers (33, 71)
mountain of educational praxis (28, 29)
mutual respect (160)
mutual working together (160)
myth
that doctors sell to themselves (44)
of measurement (119, 123, 181)

national standards (8, 179)
nature/nurture debate (85)
needs of society (82, 144)
New Testament (205)

off the record (177, 182, 183)
ontology / ontological / ontologically (48, 51, 139, 155)

paragraphs, four important (71)
patient/ patients
care (3, 6, 7, 8, 9, 21-5, 30, 37, 56, 139, 141, 143, 148, 152, 168, 191, 202)
quality and safety of (141)
role (17)
personal
philosophy (34, 35, 39, 63, 79, 91)
qualities (6, 35, 50, 80, 83, 85, 86, 93, 98, 99, 111)
personality and character (86, 92)
personhood (50, 52, 69, 139, 142)
philosophy of practice (70)
philosophy as useful to teachers (109)
phronesis (40)
phronimon (98)
Planning
aims and intentions (82)
and preparing for teaching (145)
design of small educational activities (176)
for teaching (13)
meticulous (143)
some important issues (145)
poetry (37)
portfolio
evidence (37)
ideas for the future (199)
patterns of achievement (125)

Postgraduate Certificate (PG Cert) (14, 18, 24, 37, 63, 77, 91, 133, 159, 175, 201)
postgraduate medical education
    a serious challenge to (3)
Positive personal relationships (7)
PowerPoint presentations (34, 88)
practical reasoning (9, 25, 28, 35, 39, 41, 55, 137, 151, 153)
practice
    clarifying the term (45-6)
    community of (49)
    modes of (59-60, 69-71)
    nature of educational (56-7)
    nature of medical (53-6)
    professional (46-7)
    ribal conceptions of (50-3)
    theorized (109)
    traditions of (47-8)
    values that shape (57)
practicing interpretively (55, 169)
praxis (27, 28, 29, 33-41, 55, 111, 116, 117, 137, 158, 171, 201)
    definition (35, 40)
    praxis in action (201)
principles of procedure (89)
professional
    conversation (see conversation)
    practice (5, 8, 21, 25, 41, 43-7, 50, 51, 54, 57, 58, 59, 60, 63, 65, 75, 85, 97, 99, 101, 106, 115, 127, 129, 130, 138, 157, 172, 198)
    practice, nature of (5, 8, 44, 50, 75, 129, 157, 198)
    judgement, assessment of (122)
professionalism (23, 46-7, 60, 98, 110, 114, 120, 127, 129-30, 132, 145, 160, 191)
protocol /s (4, 5, 19, 28, 30, 40, 41, 46, 51, 52, 56, 59, 60, 65-7, 80, 92, 105, 132, 147)

Quality Assurance (75, 156)
qualities
    of character or personality (99)
    personal (6, 35, 80, 83, 85, 86, 93, 98, 99)
    qualities, teacherly (72)
quality
    and use of informal formative assessment (175, 186)
    educational (21, 171)
    of teaching and learning (156)

Readership (of the book) (8)
reflection
    as a central means of learning (170)
    clinical (115, 116, 173, 199)
    definition of (115)
    enables learner to... (171)
    focused (97)
    literature on, as central to learning (112)
    resources for clinical (115)
    the role of The Arts in (173)
    why it matters (115)

reflection-in-action (115, 153)
reflection-on-action (115)
reflective practice (116, 171, 172, 199)
    defining characteristics of (172)
    is allied to praxis (116)
reflective writing, clinical (CRW) (115, 117, 173, 191, 197)
reflecting on and evaluating the teaching / learning process (147, 155-6)
relating teaching to learning: influential factors (187)
report
    formal on learner's achievement (177)
resource based learning (144, 153, 162, 163, 164)
resources, educational (156, 162)
resources for informal assessment (184-186)
rigourous, definition of (117)

Sabre-tooth curriculum (48)
sensitivity to words (101, 102)
serving the learner (142, 160)
social model of education (85)
Socrates (70)
Studying the learner (82, 91, 159)
Supervision, continuous daily (140)
Supervisor, educational and clinical (138)

talk and talking for learning (164)
    power of (165)
    presentation or exposition (164)
    question and answer (164)
    summarizing and meaning-making (169)
    teacher's talk (114)
    using talk for collective thinking (168)
    using talk for developing thinking (166)
teaching, learning and assessing practising doctors (8)
teaching
    as a profession (37)
    enhanced (13, 22-5, 27, 33, 35, 39, 41)
    the ordinary (147)
    three models of (108, 148, 149)
    transmission (93, 150)
teachers
    as educators (66, 89)
    as trainers (64)
    roles they can adopt (68)
    wise (see wise)
teaching
    conception of (70, 139)
telos (40)
techné (40)
theoretical
    basis of this book (111)
    studies (35, 37)
    understanding (34, 35, 39, 86)
theoria (40, 41, 108)
thinking like an educator (9, 133, 138, 143, 147)
thinking like a teacher (17, 29, 34, 38, 39)

methods and content (147)
tips for teachers (9, 29, 31, 32, 38, 39, 63, 138)
Tools of the Trade (120, 131, 132, 183, 188-91) (see also DOPs. C-bD, MiniCEX)
tradition/s of practice (47)
training programmes (21)
Training the Trainers (14, 15, 20, 21, 29-31, 37-9)
trust/trusting/trustworthy (4, 54, 63, 75, 98, 160, 179, 182, 187, 205)
truth (40, 73, 103, 108)
turning training into education (151)

Validity
    Intersubjective (105)
Values (3, 45-7, 56-9, 64, 67-8, 81, 83, 85, 88-9, 95, 98, 100-01, 107-11, 116-19, 125,129, 130, 139)
    Christian (72, 127)
    definition (57)
    educational (6, 9, 16, 22, 24, 39-41, 52, 56-8, 79, 138, 157)
    espoused educational values (58, 157)
    exploring educational values (138)
    Importance of (57, 130)
    In action (23)
    professional values (7, 57, 58, 70, 85, 125, 130, 143, 157)
    shared (25)
    values-based (34, 56-7, 105, 108, 124, 141, 157, 171, 181)
    values-in-use (58, 157, 172)
Venetian Justification (105)
virtue/s (33, 58, 72, 81, 87-8, 98-101, 139, 142, 202)
    Aristotelian (127)
    Christian (65)
    Thomist (72, 86)
    virtues-based (86, 112, 127)
virtuous ends (86)
vision (25, 27, 35-6, 53, 80, 116-7, 139, 157, 171, 172)

wants and need/s (35, 95, 141)
wise teacher (97, 142, 160)